Current Topics in Pathology
78

Ovarian Pathology

Contributors

L.L. Adcock · I. Damjanov · L.P. Dehner
H. Fox · C. Nuñez · E. Saksela
S.G. Silverberg · H.-E. Stegner

Editor

Francisco Nogales

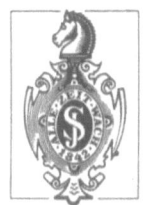

Springer-Verlag
Berlin Heidelberg New York
London Paris Tokyo

F. NOGALES, Professor Dr., Catedrático de Anatomia Patológica,
Universidad de Granada, Facultad de Medicina,
Avda. de Madrid s/n, 18012 Granada, Spain

C.L. BERRY, Professor Dr., Department of Morbid Anatomy,
The London Hospital Medical College, Whitechapel,
London E1 1BB, Great Britain

E. GRUNDMANN, Professor Dr., Gerhard-Domagk-Institut für
Pathologie der Universität, Domagkstraße 17, 4400 Münster, FRG

With 62 Figures, Some in Colour

ISBN-13: 978-3-642-74013-8   e-ISBN-13: 978-3-642-74011-4
DOI: 10.1007/978-3-642-74011-4

© Springer-Verlag Berlin Heidelberg 1989
Softcover reprint of the hardcover 1st edition 1989

Typesetting, printing and bookbinding: Universitätsdruckerei H. Stürtz AG, D-8700 Würzburg
2122/3130-543210 − Printed on acid-free paper

List of Contributors

ADCOCK, L.L., Dr., Associate Professor — Department of Obstetrics and Gynecology (Division of Gynecologic Oncology), University of Minnesota Medical School, Minneapolis, MN 55455, USA

DAMJANOV, I., Prof., Dr. — Department of Pathology, Thomas Jefferson University, Jefferson Medical College, Philadelphia, PA 19107, USA

DEHNER, L.P., Prof., Dr. — Department of Laboratory Medicine and Pathology (Division of Surgical Pathology), University of Minnesota Medical School, Minneapolis, MN 55455, USA

FOX, H., Prof. Dr., F.R.C. Path., F.R.C.O.G. — Department of Pathology, University of Manchester, Stopford Building, Manchester M13 9PL, Great Britain

NUÑEZ, C., Dr., F.I.A.C., Director — Cytopathology Laboratory, The Cleveland Clinic Foundation, Cleveland, OH 44106, USA

SAKSELA, E., Prof., Dr. — Department of Pathology, University of Helsinki, Haartmaninkatu 3, SF-00290 Helsinki, Finland

SILVERBERG, S.G., Prof., Dr. — Department of Pathology, George Washington University, Medical Center, 2300 Eye St., N.W., Washington, D.C. 20037, USA

STEGNER, H.-E., Prof., Dr. — Department of Pathology, University of Hamburg, University Hospital of Eppendorf, Martinistr. 52, 2000 Hamburg 20, FRG

Preface

When presented with the task of editing a volume on such a wide and diverse topic as Ovarian Pathology, it is difficult to know how to limit the range of subjects to be covered when there are so many taxonomical entities, both neoplastic and reactive that could be included. However, I have chosen to cover concepts that are not usually dealt with in depth in Gynaecological Pathology textbooks.

From the clinicopathological viewpoint, a wealth of new data has been updated and critically reappraised. As patient prognosis and treatment should always be our first concern, I have made the nucleus of this book five chapters which offer a structured valouration of ovarian neoplasms aiming for a better understanding between pathologist and oncologist, especially when dealing with staging ovarian tumours. This is of particular relevance as, until now, tumour stage seems to be the most important parameter in predicting the outcome and treatment of ovarian tumours. However, reliable staging procedures are frequently ignored by gynaecologists whilst histopathologists often seem to play a non-specified role, largely disconnected from the clinical picture. Here, L.L. ADCOCK and L.P. DEHNER provide a rationale to serve as a basis for greater clarity and interspeciality understanding of the staging of ovarian tumours whilst C. NUÑEZ considers the role of cytopathology and fine needle aspiration as non- or minimally invasive techniques in staging and management.

Although histopathological assessment of differentiation is playing an increasingly important part in the prognosis of breast and prostate tumours, its value in ovarian tumours is still unclear and S.G. SILVERBERG reviews in depth this controversial problem. The until recently rigid concept of borderline tumours is critically reconsidered and the important recent progress made in this field reported by H. FOX. E. SAKSELA reviews in detail the immunohistochemistry of ovarian tumours and emphasizes how this is becoming an increasingly significant adjunct of both clinical and histopathological concepts.

I have also included a chapter dealing with non-neoplastic pathology of the ovary, namely a systematic review of hormonally reactive conditions by H.-E. STEGNER.

The chapter dealing with experimental neoplasms, clearly explained by I. DAMJANOV, provides both the pathologist and clinician with a fresh insight into concepts only normally found in experimental journals.

I would like to take this opportunity to thank my wife, H.R.
NOGALES, M.B. Ch.B., for her assistance in preparing this edition, M.C.
SANTOS and J. GARRIDO for their secretarial help and H. HERION, W.
BERGSTEDT and U.S. DAVIS of Springer-Verlag, Heidelberg, for their
patience and co-operation.

Granada   FRANCISCO NOGALES

Contents

Indexed in ISR

Ovarian Tumours in Laboratory and Domestic Animals

I. DAMJANOV

Introduction

In contrast with the relatively high incidence of human ovarian tumours, spontaneous tumours occur seldom in the ovaries of other mammals. However, despite their relative rarity, ovarian neoplasms of common laboratory and domestic animals have received considerable attention and have been investigated from many aspects in an attempt to develop laboratory models for the study of etiology, histogenesis and the response to therapy of equivalent human tumours. Experimental tumours can be induced readily in the ovaries by several methods and are even more suitable for laboratory studies.

Ovarian tumours in laboratory and domestic animals fall into three categories: tumours of surface mesothelium, also known as germinal (coelomic) epithelium; sex cord tumours; and germ cell tumours. These are mostly comparable to their human counterparts (LINGEMAN 1974; NIELSEN et al. 1976; CARTER and IRD 1976; LEMON and GUBAREVA 1977). However, certain human ovarian tumours such as e.g. Brenner tumours, clear cell carcinoma or endometrioid tumours have not been recorded in animals. Also, there is no consensus whether tubular adenomas of rodents (LINGEMAN 1974) or domestic animals (NORRIS et al. 1969b; 1970) represent Sertoli cell tumours or just a histological variant of granulosa cell tumours.

1 Tumours of Surface Epithelium

Epithelial tumours originating from the surface mesothelium i.e. coelemic epithelial covering of the ovary occur spontaneously in mice (SLYE et al. 1920), rats

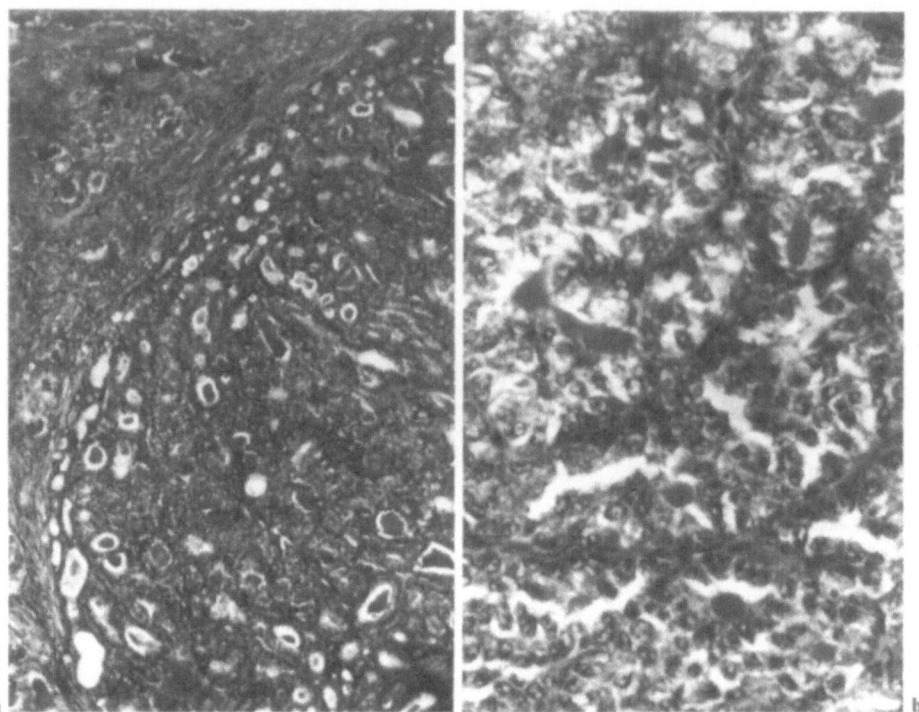

Fig. 1 a, b. Ovarian adenocarcinoma of a domestic hen. **a** × 90; **b** × 280

(Snell 1965), dogs (Nielsen et al. 1976) and hens (Fredrickson 1987). Tumours are arbitrarily divided into adenomas and adenocarcinomas, but the histological distinction of benign from malignant lesions is not always clear cut. Descriptive adjectives such as papillary serous or cystic are used for some of these tumours to denote their gross or microscopic appearance and emphasize their similarity to human tumours.

Mouse tumours originating from the surface epithelium are quite rare. Slye et al. (1920) autopsied 22,000 mice and found 44 ovarian tumours, 38 of which were classified as benign papillary adenomas. Rat cystadenocarcinomas, capable of abdominal dissemination are also rare (Crain 1958). The Registry of Experimental Cancer of the National Cancer Institute, Bethesda, Maryland listed 2 spontaneous epithelial mouse and 5 rat tumours of the ovary classified as cystadenoma or cystadenocarcinoma (Lingeman 1974). Interestingly, one of these rat tumours that metastasized throughout the abdominal cavity also contained foci of malignant cartilage in the stroma, suggesting that it might have been a carcinosarcoma.

Serous papillary adenomas and adenocarcinomas are relatively common in dogs (Nielsen et al. 1976). Like human equivalents, these tumours usually form cystic, fluid filled cavities lined by serous cuboidal cells. Bilateral tumours and peritoneal metastases are likewise common. In the absence of metastasis diagnosis of malignancy may be rather arbitrary and is based on the assessment of the size of the tumour, invasion of the ovarian stroma and the mitotic activity (NIELSEN et al. 1976).

Ovarian epithelial tumours occur frequently in domestic hens (FREDRICKSON 1987). Although there are no statistical data on the incidence of such tumours, the general consensus of avian pathologists is that ovarian adenocarcinomas represent the most common forms of poultry neoplasia. Best and most complete data stem from the longitudinal study performed by FREDRICKSON (1987) at the University of Connecticut that included 466 hens followed for $3^1/_2$ years. An amazing number of animals, corresponding to 32% of all hens, developed ovarian tumours. An additional 8% of the hens had oviductal tumours and 5% had leiomyomas of the suspending ligament of the oviduct thus bringing the incidence of genital tumours to 45%. Most ovarian tumours (24%) were of epithelial origin and were classified as adenocarcinomas (Fig. 1). Typically tumours formed papillary excrescences, invaded and destroyed the ovary and spread over the serosal surfaces of the adjacent organs. Implantation on the surface of distant abdominal organs and ascites, amounting up to 500 ml were found in some cases. Hematogeneous metastases outside of the abdominal cavity did not occur. There was no evidence of viral infection or hormonal disbalance that could account for such a high incidence of tumours in these hens.

2 Sex Cord Tumours

Granulosa cell tumours either pure or mixed with so-called tubular adenomas or theca cell components represent the most common spontaneous ovarian tumour in laboratory animals LINGEMAN 1974; FIRTH et al. 1981). Approximately one third of all Osborne-Mendel rats develop granulosa cell tumours with age (LINGEMAN 1974). Spontaneous granulosa cell tumours of mice are common in older animals. However, in strain SWR mice, which have a genetic predisposition malignant granulosa cell tumours develop at an early age (BEAMER et al. 1985). Maternally transmitted susceptibility leads to the formation of granulosa cell tumours as early as 4–6 weeks of age with a peak at 10 weeks. While in inbred SWR/J or SWR/Bm the incidence of granulosa cell tumours is 2.5–3.5% in some recombinant inbred mice lines it may be as high as 15%. Genetically predetermined granulosa cell tumours of SWR mice evolve simultaneously in multiple ova containing ovarian follicles of pubertal females (BEAMER et al. 1985). These tumours differ in this respect from the common granulosa cell tumours of aging rodents, which arise usually from follicles devoid of viable ova. Experimental destruction of oocytes by x-irradiation (GUTHRIE 1958), carcinogens (MARCHANT 1960) alone or combined with intrasplenic transplantation of ovaries (ARMUTH and BERENBLUM 1979) is usually accompanied by an increased incidence of ovarian granulosa cell tumours. Approximately one-half of all x-ray induced tumours are retransplantable (FURTH 1946), while the genetically predetermined tumours of SWR mice seem to be even more amenable to transplantation (BEAMER et al. 1985).

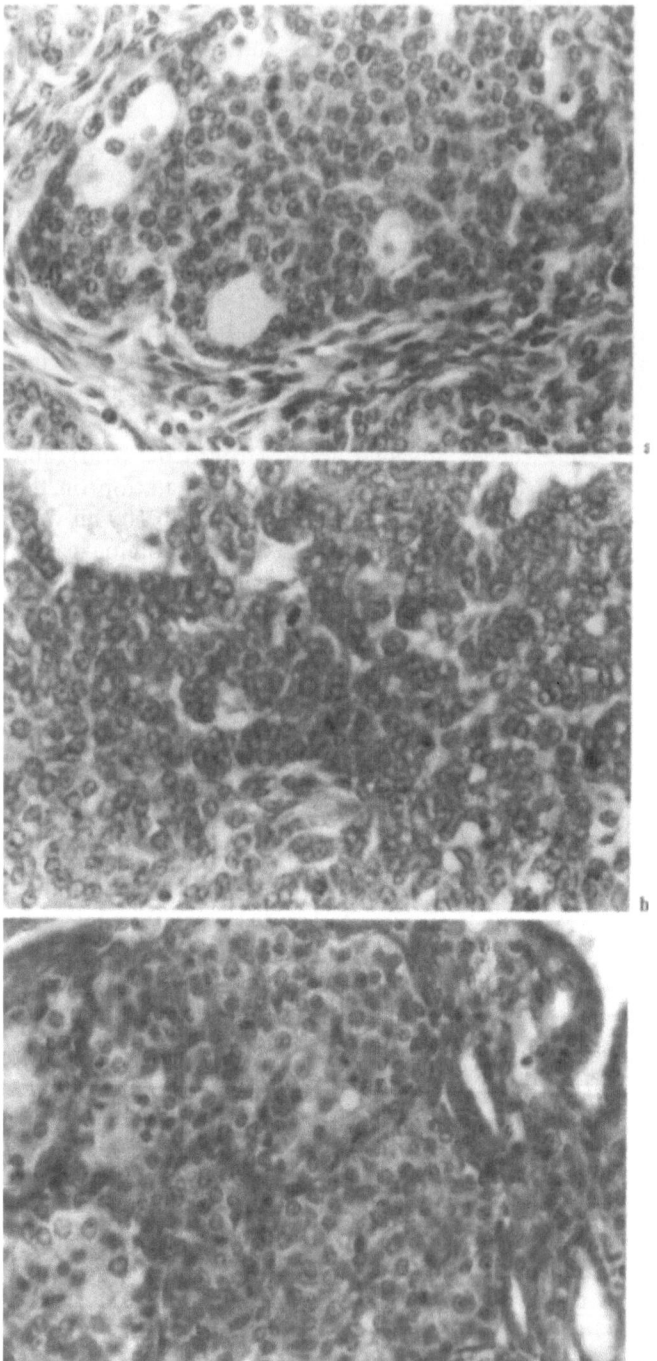

Fig. 2a–c. Ovarian granulosa cell tumour of SWR/J mice. **a** Folliculoid pattern with Call-Exner-like structures, ×280. **b** Granulosa cells arranged in sheets and ribbons. Note mitotic figures, ×280. **c** Luteinized portion of a granulosa cell tumour, ×280

Ovarian granulosa cell tumours develop spontaneously at the time of puberty in approximately 5% of inbred SWXJ-9 mice (BEAMER et al. 1988). The murine tumours show a striking resemblance to human juvenile granulosa cell tumours of the ovary in that they occur prior to adulthood, histologically show the same features and are associated with disturbed endocrine activity. Murine tumours have a definitive malignant potential.

The administration of dehydroepiandrosterone will increase eight times the incidence of granulosa cell tumours. Testosterone will also increase the incidence of such tumours whereas dehydrotestosterone is without obvious effect and 17-beta estradiol has an inhibitory effect (BEAMER et al. 1988).

Granulosa cell tumours of rodents occur in several histological forms (Fig. 2). Although the cells always show typical features of normal granulosa cells, they may grow in solid sheets, form follicle like aggregates, glandular or glomeruloid structures and even Call-Exner like rosettes (CARTER and IRD 1976; LEMON and GUBAREVA 1979). Mixed stromal-epithelial tumours may also occur (POUR 1986).

Luteinization of granulosa cells or adjacent theca and other stromal cells is quite common, contributing most likely to the hormonal activity of these neoplasms (CARTER and IRD 1976).

Canine granulosa cell tumours are as common as epithelial neoplasms in this species (NIELSEN et al. 1976). Histologically similar tumours are found in cats, mares, queens, ewes and sows (NORRIS et al. 1968; 1969a and b, 1970). Tumours may be hormonally active or inactive. The former secrete either estrogens or androgenes or both. Histologically tumours present in a sarcomatoid or folliculoid pattern. Tubular adenoma pattern is seen in some tumours classified by NORRIS et al. (1969; 1970) as Sertoli cell tumours. However, there is no universal consensus as to whether the tubule forming cells are indeed Sertoli cells or only morphological variants of granulosa cells (COTCHIN 1961).

3 Germ Cell Tumours

Spontaneous germ cell tumours have been recorded in the ovaries of mice, rats, guinea pigs, bitches, cows, cats and some other animals (DEHNER et al., 1970; DAMJANOV and SOLTER 1974; STEVENS and VARNUM 1974). Histologically, these tumours are classified as dysgerminomas, teratomas, teratocarcinomas or yolk sac carcinomas. Overall, the tumours are comparable to those seen in the human ovary.

3.1 Dysgerminoma

Dysgerminomas are most commonly found in adult or old cats and dogs (ANDREWS et al. 1974; NIELSEN et al. 1976). The tumours are composed of large polygonal cells arranged in cords and nests surrounded by connective tissue septa, sparsely infiltrated with lymphocytes. Histologically tumours resemble

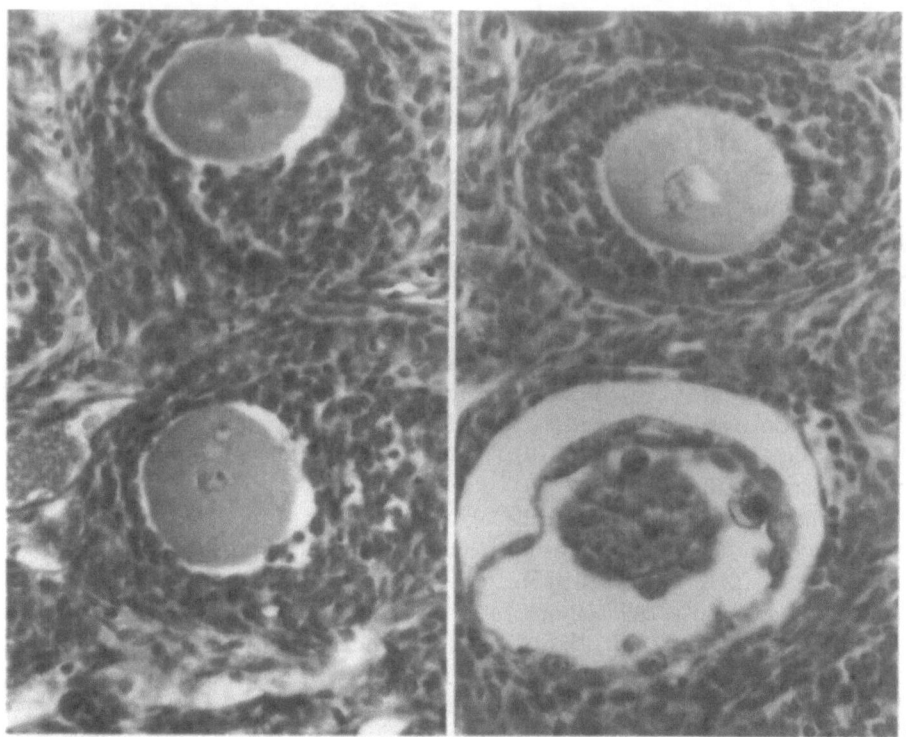

Fig. 3a, b. Ovaries of LT mice showing parthenogenetic activation of germ cells. **a** Activated oocyte (*lower*) contains two nuclei, ×280. **b** Parthenote in the blastocyst stage of embryonic development, ×280

seminomas of the testicle (NIELSEN et al. 1976) and are likewise sensitive to x-ray radiation.

3.2 Teratomas

Benign and malignant teratomas (teratocarcinomas) are rare in all laboratory animals. Only a few spontaneous tumours have been reported in mice (FAWCETT 1950; FEKETE and FERRIGNO 1952) before STEVENS and VARNUM (1974) reported that teratomas occur at an extremely high rate in inbred mice of the LT strain. Approximately 50% of all three month old mice have ovarian teratomas, many of them bilaterally. Tumours originate from parthenogenetically activated oocytes (Fig. 3). By the time of weaning, essentially all ovaries contain activated ova or parthenotes in early stages of embryogenesis. It has been shown that the parthenotes develop normally through early stages of embryogenesis corresponding to morula and blastocyst (STEVENS and VARNUM 1974; DAMJANOV et al. 1976). However, primordial germ layer formation does not occur normally and the entire growth becomes disorganized thereafter. Most tumours are benign (Fig. 4). Malignant tumours, teratocarcinomas, proved to be retransplantable

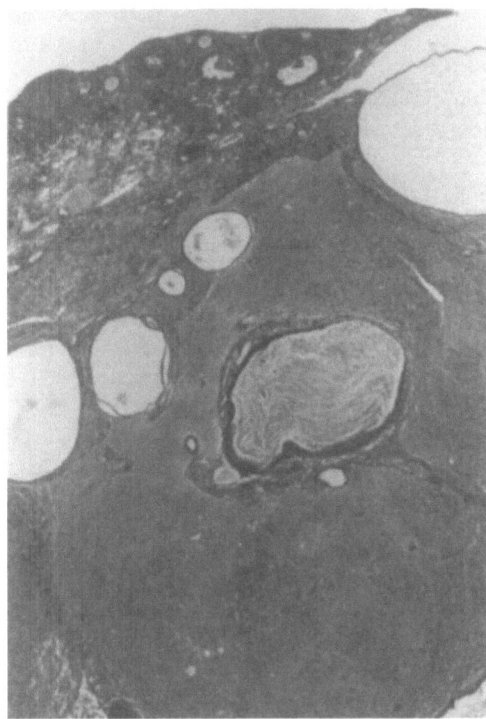

Fig. 4. Benign teratoma in the ovary of a LT mouse. The remaining ovarian tissue is in the upper portion of the photograph, ×90

and are in essence indistinguishable from testicular or embryo-derived teratocarcinomas (SOLTER and DAMJANOV 1979).

3.3 Yolk Sac Carcinomas

Essentially all yolk sac tumours discovered in murine ovaries present histologically in the parietal yolk sac (PYS) pattern (STEWART et al. 1984). PYS carcinoma cells are highly specialized, well differentiated cells surrounded by abundant extracellular matrix (PIERCE et al. 1962). These cells correspond to the parietal endoderm layer of the choriovitelline component of the placenta and the basement membrane material corresponds to the so-called Reichert's membrane that separates the embryo from trophoblastic cells and decidua.

Like the teratomas, PYS carcinomas are most probably of parthenogenetic origin. One could hypothesize that the parthenogenetically activated ova give rise to early embryonic and extraembryonic structures and that PYS carcinomas develops in such intraovarian tumours from the extraembryonic membranes known to be prone to malignant transformation (DAMJANOV and SOLTER 1974; WEWER 1982; SOBIS et al. 1983). Thus, spontaneous PYS carcinomas are nothing but clonal outgrowth of the most malignant component in teratomas (DAMJANOV 1980). In most instances all other tissues are obliterated by the PYS carci-

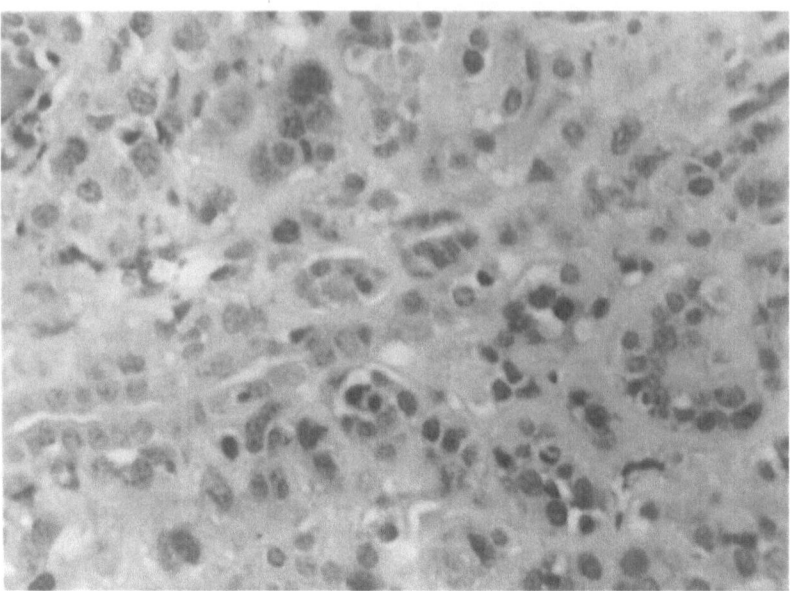

Fig. 5. Parietal yolk sac carcinoma. Note abundant extracellular basement membrane-like material, × 280

noma and the teratomatous nature of the tumours cannot be demonstrated unequivocally (Damjanov et al. 1977).

Mouse PYS carcinomas produce large amounts of basement membrane material (Fig. 5) which is only occasionally seen in human tumours so abundantly (Damjanov et al. 1984). In contrast to mouse tumours, rat yolk sac carcinomas are more often composed of both visceral and parietal yolk sac cells (Damjanov 1980; Sobis et al. 1982) and are therefore much better replicas of the human tumour.

Mouse PYS have been extensively used in biochemical studies of basement membranes (Pierce and Nakane 1967). Some major components of extracellular matrix such as laminin and entactin have been isolated from PYS tumours (Timpl et al. 1979; Chung et al. 1977; Wewer et al. 1981).

4 Conclusions

Due to the predominantly anthropocentric nature of biomedical research, most studies on animals ovarian tumours have been performed with the ultimate goal of developing new models for the better understanding of human ovarian tumours. In many instances such as parallel has been well taken and the studies were most productive. Mouse teratomas and teratocarcinomas and adenocarcinomas of hens are remarkably good replicas of their human tumour counterparts and the results from these systems could be directly relevant for human pathology. Other tumours are less acceptable surrogates.

Apart from these utilitarian concerns it is still important to know that such tumour models exist and that data from these studies could have implications for cell biology in general and human biomedical problems in particular.

Acknowledgements. Secretarial assistance of Ms. ROCHELLE HUDSON is greatly appreciated. Drs. L.C. STEVENS, W.G. BEAMER and T.N. FREDRICKSON provided some of the tumour slides photographed for this article. Original work in the author's laboratory was supported by grants from the National Institutes of Health, Bethesda, Maryland, and the W.W. Smith Charitable Fund.

References

Andrews EJ, Stookey JL, Helland DR, Slaughter LJ (1974) A histopathological study of canine and feline ovarian dysgerminomas. Canad J Comp Pathol 38:85–89

Armuth V, Berenblum I (1979) Mechanism of ovarian carcinogenesis: Effect of 7,12-dimethyl-benza (a) anthracene administration of intrasplenic ovarian grafts in unilaterally ovariectomized C3HeB/ Fe mice. J Natl Cancer Inst 63:1047–1050

Beamer WG, Hoppe PC, Whitten WK (1985) Spontaneous malignant granulosa cell tumors in ovaries of young SWR mice. Cancer Res 45:5575–5581

Beamer WG, Shultz KL, Tennent BJ (1988) Induction of ovarian granulosa cell tumors in SWXJ-9 mice with dehydroepiandrosterone. Cancer Res 49:2788–2792

Carter RL (1968) Pathology of ovarian neoplasms in rats and mice. Eur J Cancer 3:537–543

Carter RL, Ird EA (1976) Tumors of the ovary. In Pathology of Tumours in Laboratory Animals, Ed. V.S. Turusov, vol 1, part 2, pp 189–200. International Agency for Research on Cancer, Lyon

Chung AE, Freeman IL, Braginski JE, (1977) A novel extracellular membrane elaborated by a mouse embryonal carcinoma-derived cell line. Biochem Biophys Res Commun 79:859–868

Cotchin E (1961) Canine ovarian neoplasms. Rev Vet Sci 2:133–142

Crain RC (1958) Spontaneous tumors in the Rochester strain of the Wistar rat. Amer J Pathol 34:311–335

Damjanov I (1980) Parieto-visceral yolk sac carcinoma in the rat. Amer J Pathol 98:569–572

Damjanov I, Amenta PS, Zarghami F (1984) Transformation of an AFP positive yolk sac carcinoma into an AFP-negative neoplasm. Cancer 53:1902–1907

Damjanov I, Katić V, Stevens LC (1976) Ultrastructure of ovaria teratomas in LT mice. Z Krebs- forsch 83:261–267

Damjanov I, Škreb N, Sell S (1977) Origin of embryo-derived yolk sac carcinoma. Int J Cancer 19:526–530

Damjanov I, Solter D (1973) Yolk-sac carcinoma grown from explanted mouse egg cylinder. Arch Pathol 95:182–184

Damjanov I, Solter D (1974) Experimental teratoma. Curr Topics Pathol 59:69–130

Dehner LP, Norris HJ, Garner FM, Taylor HB (1970) Comparative pathology of ovarian neoplasms. III. Germ cell tumors of canine, bovine, feline, rodent and human species. J Comp Pathol 80:299– 306

Fawcett DW (1950) Bilateral ovarian teratomas in a mouse. Cancer Res 10:705–707

Fekete E, Ferrigno MA (1952) Studies on a transplantable teratoma of the mouse. Cancer Res 12:438–440

Firth CH, Zuna RE, Morgan KA (1981) A morphologic classification and incidence of spontaneous ovarian neoplasms in three inbred strains of mice. J Natl Cancer Inst 67:693–702

Fredrickson TN (1987) Ovarian tumors of the hen. Env Health Persp 73:35–51

Furth J (1949) Transplantability of induced granulosa cell tumors and of luteoma in mice. Secondary effects of these growths. Proc Soc Exp Biol Med 61:212–214

Guthrie MJ (1958) Tumorigenesis in the ovaries of mice after X-irradiation. Cancer 11:1226–1235

Lemon PG, Gubareva AV (1977) Tumours of the ovary. In: Pathology of Tumours in Laboratory Animals, Ed. VS Turusov, vol. 2, pp 385–410, International Agency for Research on Cancer, Lyon

Lingeman CH (1974) Etiology of cancer of the human ovary: A review. J Natl Cancer Inst 53:1603– 1618

Marchant J (1960) The development of ovarian tumors in ovaries grafted from mice pretreated with dimethylbenzanthracene. Inhibition by the presence of normal ovarian tissue. Brit J Cancer 14:514–518

Nielsen SW, Misdorp W, McEntee K (1976) XV. Tumours of the ovary. Bull World Health Organ 53:203–215

Norris HJ, Taylor HB, Garner FM (1968) Equine ovarian granulosa tumors. Vet Rec 82:419–420

Norris HJ, Garner FM, Taylor HB (1969a) Pathology of feline ovarian neoplasms. J Pathol 97:138–143

Norris HJ, Taylor HB, Garner FM (1969b) Comparative pathology of ovarian neoplasms. II. Gonadal stromal tumors of bovine species. Pathol Vet 6:45–58

Norris HJ, Garner FM, Taylor HB (1970) Comparative pathology of ovarian neoplasms IV. Gonadal stromal tumors of canine species. J Comp Pathol 80:399–405

Pierce GB, Midgley AR, Sri Ram J, Feldman JD (1962) Parietal yolk sac carcinoma: clue to the histogenesis of Reichert's membrane of the mouse embryo. Amer J Pathol 41:549–557

Pierce GB, Nakane PK (1967) Antigens of epithelial basement membrane of mouse, rat, and man. Lab Invest 17:499–506

Pour PM (1986) Transplacental induction of gonadal tumors in rats by nitrosamine. Cancer Res 46:4135–4138

Slye M, Holmes HF, Wells HG (1920) Primary spontaneous tumors of the ovary in mice. Studies on the incidence and heritability of spontaneous tumors of mice. J Cancer Res 5:205–226

Snell KC (1965) Spontaneous lesions of the rat. In: Pathology of Laboratory Animals. Eds. WE Ribelin, JR McCoy, pp 241–302, CC Thomas Springfield, IL

Sobis H, Van Hove L, Vandeputte M (1982) Trophoplastic and mesenchymal structures in rat yolk sac carcinoma. Int J Cancer 29:181–186

Sobis H, Van Hove L, Vandeputte M (1983) Yolk sac carcinoma of extra-embryonic origin in the 129 Sv/Sl mouse. Int J Cancer 32:367–371

Solter D, Damjanov I (1979) Teratocarcinoma and the expression of oncodevelopmental genes. Methods Cancer Res 18:277–332

Stevens LC, Varnum DS (1974) The development of teratomas from parthenogenetically activated ovarian mouse eggs. Dev Biol 37:369–380

Stewart HL, Sass B, Deringer MK, Dunn TB, Liotta LA, Togo S (1984) Pure yolk sac carcinoma of mouse uterus: report of 8 cases. J Natl Cancer Inst 73:115–122

Timpl R, Rohde H, Robey PG, Rennard SI, Foidart J-M, Martin GR (1979) Laminin – a glycoprotein from basement membranes. J Biol Chem 254:9933–9937

Wewer U (1982) Characterization of a rat yolk sac carcinoma cell line. Dev Biol 93:416–421

Wewer U, Albrechtsen R, Ruoslahti E (1981) Laminin, a nocollageneous component of epithelial basement membranes synthesized by a rat yolk sac tumor. Cancer Res 41:1518–1524

Hormonally Related Non-Neoplastic Conditions of the Ovary

H.-E. Stegner

Introduction

There are few pathological alterations of the ovary that do not in some way influence the hormonal homeostasis either by directly affecting the compartment of steroid secreting cells or by interacting with gonadotropic hormones or ovarian steroids at various levels of the regulatory axis. Owing to their origin from a common blastema, most ovarian cells are capable of steroid biosynthesis, but there is a changing pattern of ovarian steroidogenesis and of response to gonadotropic stimulation during the different periods of female life. Similar pathogenetic stimuli may lead to different responses depending on the age and the actual structural condition of the gonads. Some of these hormonally related conditions are discussed in this chapter. Unlike true neoplasms and other pathological conditions of the ovary, there exists no clear classification of hormonally related, non-neoplastic ovarian disease. A broad spectrum of conditions with different pathogenesis and morphology will be considered in this chapter.

1 Gonadal Dysgenesis

In gonadal dysgenesis, tough strands of connective tissue (streaks) are found at the site of the ovaries. Microscopically these streaks show that there is not complete aplasia (agenesis) of the gonads, but a dysgenesis. The fibromuscular matrix resembles that of ovarian stroma. It extends in the form of a ribbon under a flat or cuboidal surface epithelium. Usually germ cells are entirely lacking although persistence of some cells is possible. The cortical zone, which is free of germ cells, adjoins a noncompact hilus zone with cavernous vessels and occasional islets of hilus (LEYDIG) cells (Fig. 1). Mesonephric remnants can frequently be demonstrated. The cause of the ovarian dysgenesis is evidently not a primary deficiency of germinal cells, but an early depletion of the gonads by rapid prenatal and postnatal germ cell degeneration owing to disturbed folliculogenesis (SINGH and CARL 1966; 1967). Orderly integration into the follicular

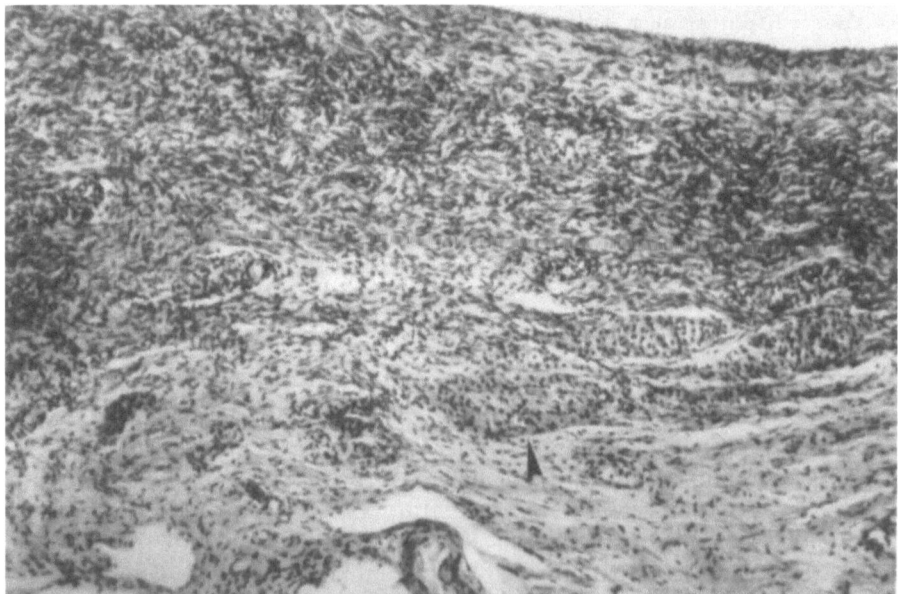

Fig. 1. Streak gonad in gonadal dysgenesis. Hilus (LEYDIG) cell complexes (*arrow*)

epithelium is the conditio sine qua non for the survival of the ovum and its transfer into the meiotic prophase.

In complete dysgenesis, all germ cells are destroyed. In incomplete gonadal dysgenesis, occasional follicles may remain and a temporary cyclic function can be maintained. There are case reports on pregnancies in ovarian dysgenesis (KING et al. 1979). Gonadal dysgenesis is found almost exclusively in genetically abnormal individuals. It is mainly associated with an anomaly of the second sex chromosome (X-chromosome monosomy). In a proportion of the cases, this is caused by a structural aberration of the second sex chromosome. In about one third of the cases, the sex chromosomal anomaly occurs as a component of a mosaic. The phenotype is a normally sized female with hypoplasia of the uterus and the breasts as well as infantile external genitalia. This is called streak gonad syndrome. Anatomically, three forms of gonadal dysgenesis are distinguished:

1) Pure gonadal dysgenesis (bilateral streaks, karyotype 46,XX: female phenotype or 46,XY; female phenotype with virilization).
2) Mixed gonadal dysgenesis (unilateral streak, contralateral testis, karyotype 46, XY or 45,X/46,XY mosaic; female phenotype with virilization).
3) Gonadal dysgenesis in combination with somatic abnormalities (bilateral streaks, karyotype mainly 45,X or 45,X/46,XY mosaics).

1.1 Pure Gonadal Dysgenesis

Karyotype 46,XX
Patients with pure gonadal dysgenesis of karyotype 46,XX are phenotypically female and of average height. The secondary sexual characteristics are not developed. Instead of the gonads, connective tissue streaks are found. As a rule, the uterus and Fallopian tubes are present but are hypoplastic. Altogether, the structure of the internal genitalia corresponds to that in TURNER's syndrome, but somatic stigmata are absent. Up to the age of puberty, development generally takes a normal course. Primary amenorrhoea and the lack of secondary sexual characteristics are the usual presenting symptoms. Endocrinologically, the 45,XX gonadal dysgenesis and the TURNER's syndrome are characterized by hypooestrinism and raised gonadotropin secretion. The 17-ketosteroids are in the lower range of normal. Phenotypically, there is no normal correlation with the chromosomal constellation in the streak syndrome. However, there are certain relations between the microscopic structure of the streak gonads and the endocrine status.

The functional activity of the dysgenetic gonads depends on the presence of steroid-active cells, i.e. cells capable of steroid hormone biosynthesis. Differentiated theca cells are necessary for oestrogen formation, progesterone is produced in the luteinized granulosa cells of the corpus luteum. Hilus (LEYDIG) cells have been identified as the site of testosterone biosynthesis under normal and pathological conditions. Ultrastructurally, all cells capable of steroid synthesis possess an identical assortment of specific organelles. Direct cell-topographic

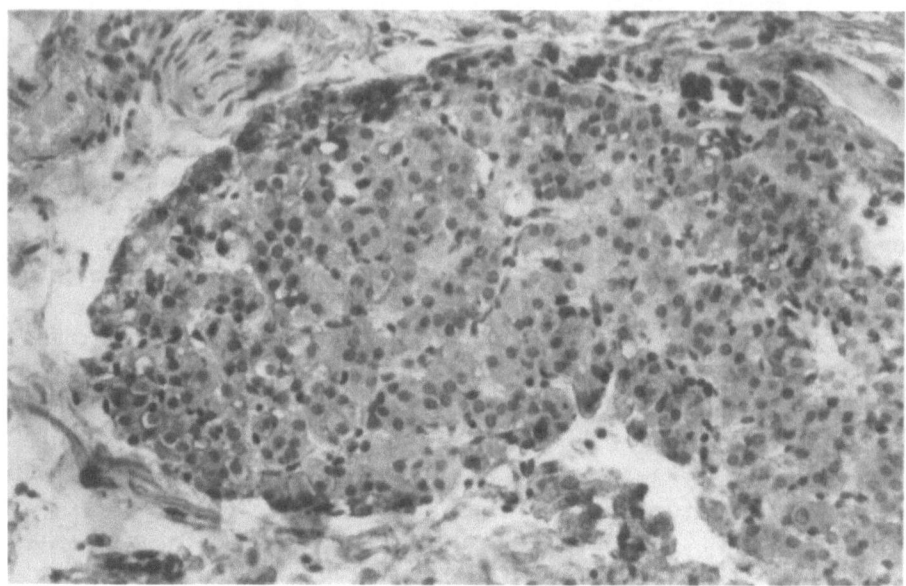

Fig. 2. Immunohistochemical demonstration of testosterone within LEYDIG cell complexes of dysgenetic gonad (46 XY dysgenesis)

detection of steroid hormones is possible by immunocytochemistry (KURMAN et al. 1978, 1981, 1984).

Immunocytochemical investigations have also shown that there is no cell specifity for the biosynthesis of the individual steroid hormones.

Streak gonads show a complete compartment of steroid-active cells only in exceptional cases of incomplete dysgenesis. In most cases, they merely have hilus (LEYDIG) cell complexes as potential sites of androgen biosynthesis (Fig. 2). This explains why virilization is found in almost 50% of the cases of pure gonadal dysgenesis. However, mixed gonadal dysgenesis – unilateral streak ovary and contralateral testis – is practically always accompanied by virilization, for function of the unilateral testis is not sufficient either to completely inhibit the development of the Mullerian derivatives or to stimulate the differentiation of the mesonephric structures and the male external genitalia (ROBBOY et al. 1982).

Karyotype 46,XX
Pure gonadal dysgenesis of 46,XY karyotype differs from the 46,XX dysgenesis in that there are more or less pronounced signs of virilization in usually tall, phenotypically female individuals. Uterus and tubes are present, epididymal structures may be detectable in the region of the streak gonads, which are free of germ cells and contain typical hilus (LEYDIG) cells singly or in groups, as well as varying amounts of tubular or follicular sex cord components. The follicular structures resemble granulosa cells, the tubular structures resemble immature SERTOLI cells. Both components show degenerative changes in the form of hyalinization or coarse calcium deposits.

The cause of aberrant testicular differentiation in 46,XY dysgenesis of male phenotype has not been completely clarified. Normal testicular development requires the presence of a functioning Y chromosome and of the histocompatibility antigen Y (H-Y antigen), a protein which binds to specific receptors of the somatic gonadal cells (WACHTEL 1979; HALL and WACHTEL 1980, HASELTINE and OHNO 1981). In the group of 46,XY dysgenesis, however, both H-Y+ and H-Y− cases are be found. According to WOLF (1979), the abnormal testicular Differentiation in the H-Y+ individuals is probably based on a defect in the gonadal receptor for H-Y antigen. A functionally inert H-Y antigen has also been proposed as a possible cause. The time and the duration of the abnormal relation determines the intersexual structural pattern of the aberrant gonads (PICKARTZ et al. 1980; MOLTZ et al. 1981). Endocrinologically, raised testosterone levels in the plasma and urine are found in 46,YX dysgenesis. The 17-ketosteroids are normal or slightly raised. The gonadotropin excretion corresponds to that of the postmenopause. The oestradiol levels are in the range of the early follicular phase.

In XY gonadal dysgenesis, there is a high risk of malignant transformation of the aberrant gonads. The most frequent tumour type is the gonadoblastoma (SCULLY 1953). This is a tumour which consist of neoplastic germ cells and undifferentiated sex cord cells of granulosa or SERTOLI cell type (SCULLY 1953, 1970; TALERMAN 1974, 1980). Macroscopically, these are small round, well delineated tumours, and rarely larger than 5 cm in diameter, but often only visible microscopically in the streak gonads (DAMJANOV and KLAUBER 1980; GUNNALA et al. 1981). The progression of the primary gonadoblastoma to dysgerminoma or combination with other highly malignant germ cell tumours (i.e. embryonal carcinoma, immature teratoma, choriocarcinoma) finally determines the prognosis (TALERMAN 1974, 1980; LUZZATTO et al. 1979; BONAKDAR and PEISNER 1980). Bilateral adnexectomy performed as early as possible is indicated in XY dysgenesis due to its tendency of malignant transformation (BARAKAT et al. 1979; WOODCOCK et al. 1979; CURTIS et al. 1980). Clinical demonstration of a tumour is not always possible before surgical removal of the gonad. A high proportion of gonadoblastomas are only discovered in histological investigation of the macroscopically normal streak gonads.

Bilateral adnexectomy is also indicated in order to eliminate the pathological androgen source, above all in mixed gonadal dysgenesis. Prepubertal surgery prevents virilization. Postpubertal surgery can reduce the extent of virilization and improve the female secondary sexual characteristics.

1.2 Mixed Gonadal Dysgenesis

In mixed gonadal dysgenesis, an asymmetric gonadal development with unilateral testis and contralateral streak gonad is found. The karyotype is 46,XY or 45X/46,XY mosaic. The phenotype is female with different degrees of virilization. Somatic malformations are not present. Diagnosis of mixed gonadal dysgenesis is not possible from the karyotype alone, but requires a histological examination of the gonads.

1.3 Gonadal Dysgenesis in Combination with Somatic Abnormalities (TURNER's Syndrome)

In the syndrome described by TURNER (1938), gonadal dysgenesis is accompanied by shortness of stature and various other somatic abnormalities. The frequency and combination of the somatic malformations are exceedingly variable. About 50% of the cases are short infantile females with a short, thick neck with pterygium and a low hairline. The thorax is broad and shieldlike. Multiple pigment naevi are found in more than 60% of the cases. Cubitus valgus and hypoplasia of the nails are present in about 50%. Congenital lymphoedema of the hands and feet in neonates can be a first indication of the genetic disorder.

The causes of the X-chromosomal monosomy in TURNER's syndrome have not been completely clarified. The disorder leading to monosomy X may occur during oogenesis or spermatogenesis, or even after fertilization. Genetic investigations suggest that the loss of the male Y chromosome is more frequent than the loss of the female X chromosome. However, more probable than a loss of the sex chromosome in meiosis by non-disjunction is a disorder of the division of the zygote occuring after fertilization, which may give rise to two or more cell lines of different constellation. Thus in women with TURNER's syndrome, 45,X/46,XY; 45,X/47,XXX; 45,X/44,XX/47,XXX as well as 45,X/46,XY and 45,X/47,XYY mosaics have been observed.

2 Gonadotropin-Resistent Ovary Syndrome

The gonadotropin-resistent ovary syndrome was first described by KINCH et al. (1963) and designated as a "follicular" form of ovarian dysgenesis. Patients affected by this syndrome present with primary or secondary amenorrhoea, and the resistance to gonadotropins may be relative rather than absolute, and sometimes only temporary (CAMPENHOUT et al. 1972; KIM 1974; DEWHURST et al. 1975). The history of apparently normal menstrual cycles prior to the onset of symptoms and a negative stimulation effect after use of exogenous gonadotropins support the notion that gonadotropin-resistant ovary syndrome is usually an acquired disorder not related to any abnormality of FSH. Moreover, antibodies to FSH have not been detected in this syndrome. An acquired defect at the level of the follicular compartment in terms of a reduced number of follicles or functional incompetence of FSH and/or LH receptors, seems to be plausible and highly probable. A congenital defect of receptors, theoretically, would prevent the normal development of secondary sex characteristics due to gonadotropin insensitivity of the steroid-producing cell compartment. The ovaries in gonadotropin-resistent ovary syndrome show morphologically normal or reduced numbers of primordial follicles (STARUP et al. 1971).

3 Premature Hypergonadotropic Ovarian Failure (Premature Menopause)

Premature ovarian failure is characterized by menarche at a normal age followed by secondary hypergonadotropic amenorrhea prior to 35 years of age, more than 15 years earlier than the average physiological menopause. In principle, premature ovarian failure can be caused by three fundamental conditions:

1) An initial low number of primordial follicles.
2) Enhanced follicular atresia at any stage prior to the expected age of menopause.
3) Postnatal destruction of oocytes by different endogenous or exogenous causes.

There are many proposed causes of premature ovarian failure, including chromosomal anomalies, infection, autoimmune disease, drugs and toxins, radiation, enzyme defects, and biological variants of hormones or their receptors.

However, the largest group of cases reported in the literature corresponds to true menopause and is characterized by total depletion of primordial follicles. Some scattered residual primary follicles or sporadic menses do not exclude the diagnosis (REBAR et al. 1983). However, the patient has irreversibly lost her reproductive capacity and needs both symptomatic and psychological support.

4 Autoimmune Ovarian Failure

An autoimmune disease process directed mainly against steroid-producing ovarian cells is suggested by several clinical and immunological observations. Initial evidence was drawn from a high association of premature ovarian failure and a variety of autoimmune disorders such as HASHIMOTO's thyroiditis, ADDISON's and BASEDOW's disease, hypoparathyroidism, rheumatoid arthritis, myasthenia gravis, juvenile diabetes mellitus, moniliasis, pernicious anemia and others. In some of these cases, anti-ovarian antibodies directed against various components of the follicular or interstitial tissue, can be demonstrated by immunofluorescent technique (DE MORAES-RUEHSEN et al. 1972; IRVINE et al. 1968, 1969). In the cases of premature menopause reported by COULAM et al. (1982) evidence of autoimmune processes was found in 18% of the patients. Furthermore, interactions between the immune system and gonadal development can be suggested from the observation that in females with congenital absence of thymus who die before puberty, no primordial follicles can be found in the ovaries. TAGUCHI et al. (1980) described a particular type of ovarian dysgenesis which develops in mice after neonatal thymectomy at the critical age of 2–4 days after birth.

5 Luteinized Unruptured Follicle syndrome (LUF)

In the so-called luteinized unruptured follicle syndrom (LUF) the follicle shows normal preovulatory enlargement but fails to release the ovum. As indicated from delayed rise of basal body temperature and slow rise of serum progesterone reaching lower-than-normal levels, the theca-granulosa cells are inadequately luteinized and the luteal phase is shortened. Sonographic monitoring of follicular growth and laparoscopic findings show that LUF may be the cause of inadequate corpus luteum function in a considerable proportion of cases of infertility (KONINCKX 1981; SCHNEIDER et al. 1983). The mechanisms leading to luteinization of the unruptured follicle are still under discussion. A number of physiologically active nonsteroidal substances (maturation inhibitor, luteinization inhibitor, inhibitory protein) secreted by the granulosa epithelium appear to act primarily within the ovary as factors controlling the granulosa cell luteinization and maturation of the oocyte and might be responsible for disturbed ovulation and inadequate corpus luteum formation (STONE et al. 1978; CHANNING et al. 1982; DI ZEREGA et al. 1982). They are being isolated at the present time and should shed new light on the local control of ovarian function.

6 Polycystic Ovarian Disease (PCOD, STEIN LEVENTHAL Syndrome)

The classical symptoms of STEIN LEVENTHAL Syndrome include oligomenorrhoea, hirsutism, infertility secondary to anovulation and palpable, enlarged multicystic ovaries. Individual presenting symptoms may vary, but taken over a large series show relative uniformity. Up to 75% of patients present with abnormal, excessive hair growth, characteristically in the facial region, the limbs and the genitals. Typically, normal menarche and initial normal menstruation are followed by oligomenorrhoea progressing to secondary amenorrhoea. If pregnancy should occur during this process, the normal cycle may be restored after delivery.

The characteristic gross changes consist of enlarged cystic ovaries. Both ovaries tend to be almost uniformly involved and resemble pubescent gonads, being 2 to 5 times the normal size.

The ovarian capsule is thick and avascular and has a pearly white appearance. Multiple subcortical follicles 2 to 10 mm in diameter are seen on cut section. Microscopically, a dense and thickened tunica albuginea is seen. The cystic follicles are densely packed and lined with a few layers of granulosa epithelium. Hyperplasia and luteinization of the theca interna is usually present and often striking. The presence of some corpora albicantia suggest that an occasional ovulation and development of corpus luteum has occured. The cortical stroma may be hyperplastic and may show islands of luteinized interstitial cells. Hilar cell nests are more frequently and larger compared with sections of normal ovaries of reproductive age.

The common findings of hirsutism in PCOD patients is a reflection of hyperandrogenism, resulting from elevation of all the androgens, including testosterone, androstenediol, dehydroepiandrosterone sulfate, and androstenedione (MAHESH and GREENBLATT 1964; DIGNAM et al. 1964; ITO and HORTON 1971; DE VANE et al. 1975). It is usually found accompanied by increased levels of LH and oestrogens and reduced FSH secretion. It has been proposed that the androgen excess accounts for the moderately elevated oestrogen (oestrone) levels through peripheral conversion of androgens to oestrogens within the extraglandular fat tissue (DE VANE et al. 1975). The oestrogen then feeds back to the hypothalamic-pituitary axis inducing inappropriate gonadotropin secretion with an elevated LH/FSH ratio; such that ovarian changes are secondary. Conversely, the ovary may be the main source of androgen excess. GOLDZIEHER and AXELROD (1963) incubated tissue from polycystic and normal ovaries with labeled precursors and demonstrated that there was only minimal production of oestrogens by the PCOD ovarian tissue and proposed that there was a deficiency of aromatase, 17-hydroxylase, and 3-beta-hydroxysteroid dehydrogenase. ERICKSON et al. (1979) reported that the aromatase activity of granulosa cells was deficient, and they attributed this to inappropriate gonadotropin stimulation rather than to the inherent (genetic) defect in the granulosa cells. Based on in vitro studies REBAR (1983) suggests that the absence of aromatase activity may be causally related to low local concentrations of FSH rather than to an intrinsic abnormality of the granulosa epithelium. In vivo administration of FSH, increases circulating E2 and E1 levels dramatically with a concurrent decrease in androgen levels indicating a rise of aromatase activity, and both clomiphene citrate (CC) and gonadotropin therapy have proven to be effective in induction of ovulation in PCOD patients as shown by several groups.

Thus it can be concluded that the hypothalamic-pituitary axis in the PCOD is functionally intact and the functional disturbances result from inappropriate oestrogen feed back; however, the primary source of the abnormal androgen production is not clear. KIRSCHNER and JACOBS (1971) found an elevated testosterone level in only the ovarian vein in most hirsute PCOD patients and in only a few was an elevated level recorded in the adrenal vein. This suggests that the androgenic source could lie in the ovaries, perhaps as a primary hyperplasia of the androgen synthesizing cells. This would explain why simple wedge resection, reducing functioning ovarian tissue, often proves an effective treatment (COHEN 1979; ADASHI et al. 1981; HJÖRTRUP et al. 1983).

7 Non-Neoplastic Functional Cysts (Retention Cysts)

Retention cysts develop by fluid accumulation within preformed cavities. According to the type of epithelium the following functional ovarian cysts can be distinguished:

– follicle cysts
– corpus luteum cysts
– theca-lutein cysts
– inclusion cysts of surface epithelium

Retention cysts are extremely common, appearing predominantly during reproductive age (functional cysts) due to disturbed gonadotropic regulation or local
causes such as chronic inflammation or postinflammatory sclerosis, but may
also be found during times of endocrinological imbalance, such as puberty
and perimenopause. Complete obliteration of the epithelial lining may result
in „simple cysts" of unknown histogenesis.

7.1 Follicular Cysts

Follicular cysts are the most commonly found functional cysts of the ovary.
They rarely exceed 5 to 6 cm in diameter, and have a smooth cut surface and
a thin wall, and usually contain clear watery fluid. They are lined by a few
layers of typical granulosa cells surrounded by a capillary rich small theca
interna (Fig. 3). Due to increasing pressure of the retained secretion the lining
may be compressed and finally obliterated, and when this occurs, differential
diagnosis with non follicular cysts becomes extremely difficult.

There is no clear distinction between Graafian follicles, persistent follicles
and small follicular cysts when only the size of the cystic lesion is considered.
According to sonographic measuring, the size of normal ovulatory follicles
ranges from 20 to 24 mm in diameter and may be somewhat greater in therapeut-
ically induced ovulation. In both preovulatory follicles and persisting follicles,

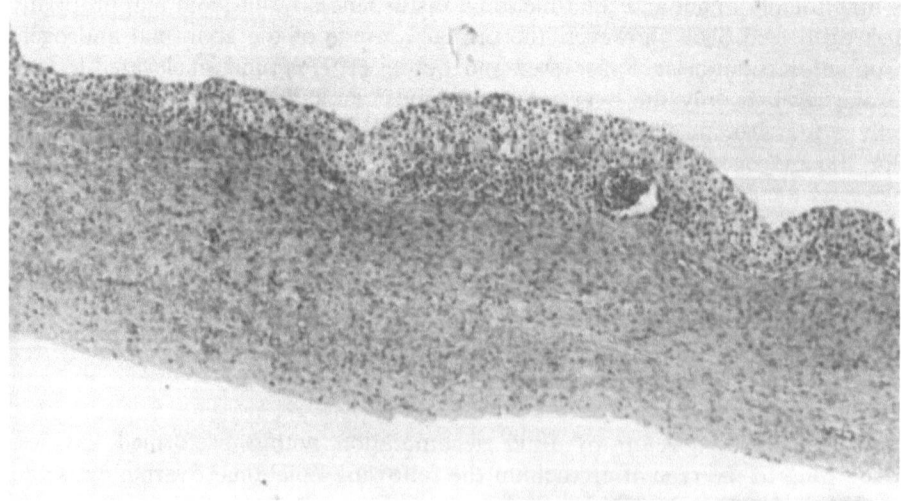

Fig. 3. Follicular cyst lined by few layers of typical granulosa cells

the ovum and granulosa cells are preserved while in follicular cysts the oocyte is degenerated and the granulosa epithelium reduced to few distorted layers or compressed to a single layer of cuboidal or flattened cells.

Follicular cysts usually undergo spontaneous involution after 2 or 3 months and young women can justifiably be kept under observation for this length of time, however, if the cysts persist, laparoscope-directed aspiration or surgical excision is indicated.

7.2 Follicular Cysts in Newborns and Infants

Advanced stages of follicular growth are generally present in all ovaries of infants and children (LINTERN-MOORE et al. 1974; PETERS 1980). The maximum diameter of antral follicles encountered routinely in the infant ovary, however, is considerably less than that of preovulatory follicles in the adult. Follicular cysts are infrequent but account for one-third to one-half of clinically significant ovarian enlargement in infants and children up to 15 years.

Follicular cysts can be a source of excessive estrogen secretion and sexual precocity in children (STEINER and HADAW 1964). In some cases precocity has

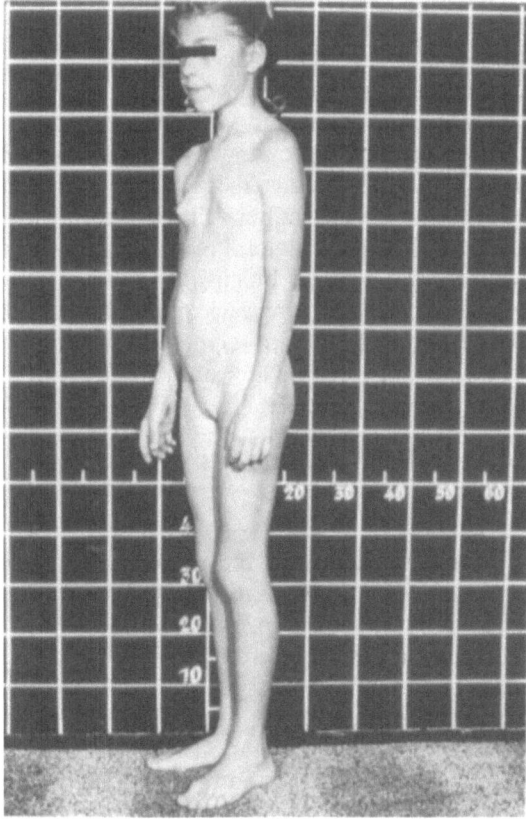

Fig. 4. Seven year-old girl with sexual precocity presenting multiple cystic follicles and unilateral follicle cyst of 7 cm in diameter

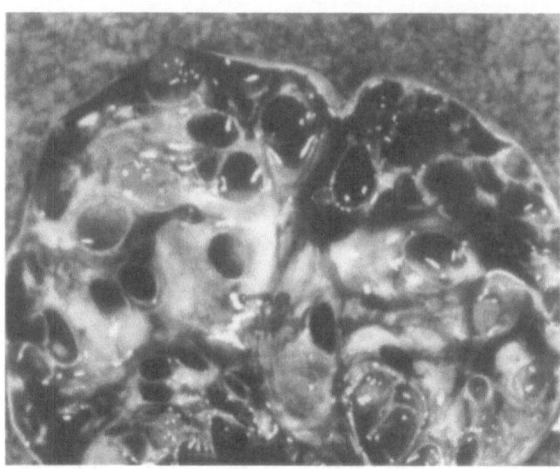

Fig. 5. Wedge resection from the ovary of a seven year old girl with sexual precocity. Numerous cystic follicles densely packed within inner and outer cortex of the ovary

been cured by removal of the cyst, indicating its lack of dependence on gonadotropic stimulation (so-called gonadal precocity: precocious pseudopuberty). Figure 4 shows a 7 years-old girl who had clinical signs of oestrogen stimulation, with many secondary sexual characteristics. Plasma gonadotropins were found within the low levels of normal infants (FSH 0.3 ng/l, LH 0,3 ng/l) and did not respond to LH-RH stimulation test. Urinary oestrogen excretion was 3 to 6 ng/24 hours, plasma oestradiol levels 9 pg/ml maximum.

The right ovary was replaced by a single follicle cyst of 7 cm in diameter. On microscopic examination the inner wall of the cyst was lined by 2 to 3 layers of granulosa cells supported by a thin fibrous theca. There were no signs of luteinization of the theca cells nor of interstitial cells. Corpora lutea or corpora albicantia could not be found. The contralateral ovary was enlarged to 4 × 4 cm due to multiple thin walled cystic follicles bulging the ovarian capsule. Histological examination of a wedge resection revealed numerous cystic follicles densely packed in the ovarian cortex but also numerous primordial ova and secondary follicles (Fig. 5). Corpora lutea or albicantia were lacking. There was no luteinization of thecal or interstitial cells.

7.3 Corpus Luteum Cysts

Persistence of corpus luteum is a common finding in the reproductive cycle of some species such as cattle and dogs. In the human, delayed regression of luteal cells results in maintenance of progesterone production and delayed menstruation mostly followed by persistent uterine bleeding. In cystic corpora lutea the inner surface of the luteal cell compartement is covered by a thin layer of fibroblasts and the cavity is filled by clear yellow fluid or blood (Fig. 6). The luteal cells are found in various stages of degeneration (Fig. 7). Corpus luteum cysts rarely exceed the size of 5 cm in diameter and they may be subject to torsion or rupture with intra-abdominal hemorrhage, simulating an ectopic pregnancy.

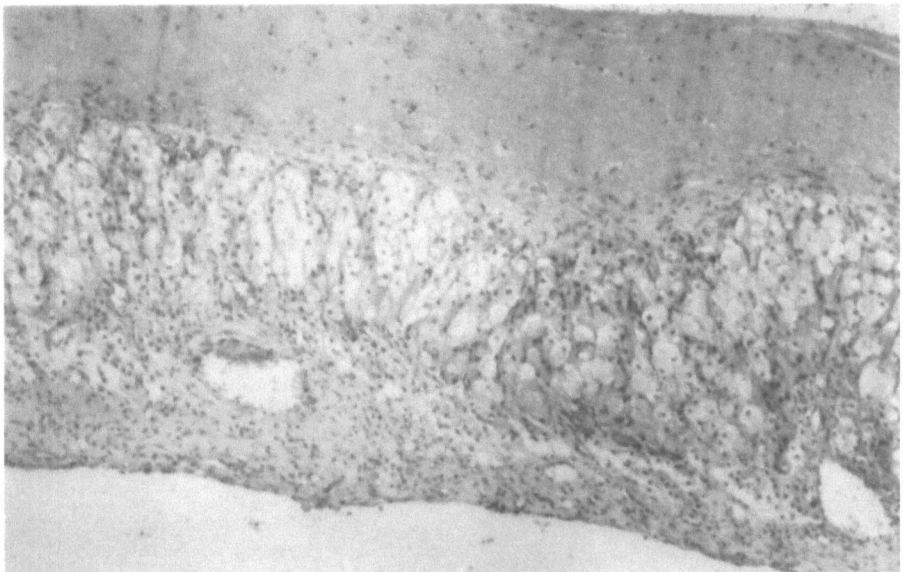

Fig. 6. Section from Corpus luteum cyst. The inner surface of the luteal cell compartement is covered by a small layer of fibroblasts

7.4 Theca Lutein Cysts

Theca lutein cysts are characterized by hyperplasia of the theca layer. Granulosa cells are reduced in number and the follicular lining may be completely atrophic (Fig. 8). Although singular theca lutein cysts may occasionally be found, they are usually multiple and involve both ovaries. They obviously result from excess stimulation of the theca interna by unusually high levels of circulating gonadotropins particularly in twin and multiple pregnancies, trophoblastic disease, and in patients receiving gonadotropin therapy for induction of ovulation. Theca lutein cysts should be differentiated from large solitary luteinized follicle cysts (CLEMENT and SCULLY 1979) in pregnant and puerperal patients. In these cases cysts are large, measuring up to 25 cm in diameter, solitary and unilocular, resembling serous cystadenomas. On microscopic examination, they are lined by single or multiple layers of luteinized cells showing focal nuclear atypia. Although different in their gross morphology and histologic appearance from theca lutein cells, both lesions seem to be pathogenetically related.

7.5 Inclusion Cysts

Inclusion cysts are non-functional cysts rarely exceeding 1–2 cm in diameter. Although they may be large enough to be detected on macroscopic examination, they more usually occur as multiple, microscopic cysts lying close to the ovarian surface, but they may also be found in the deeper layers of the cortex.

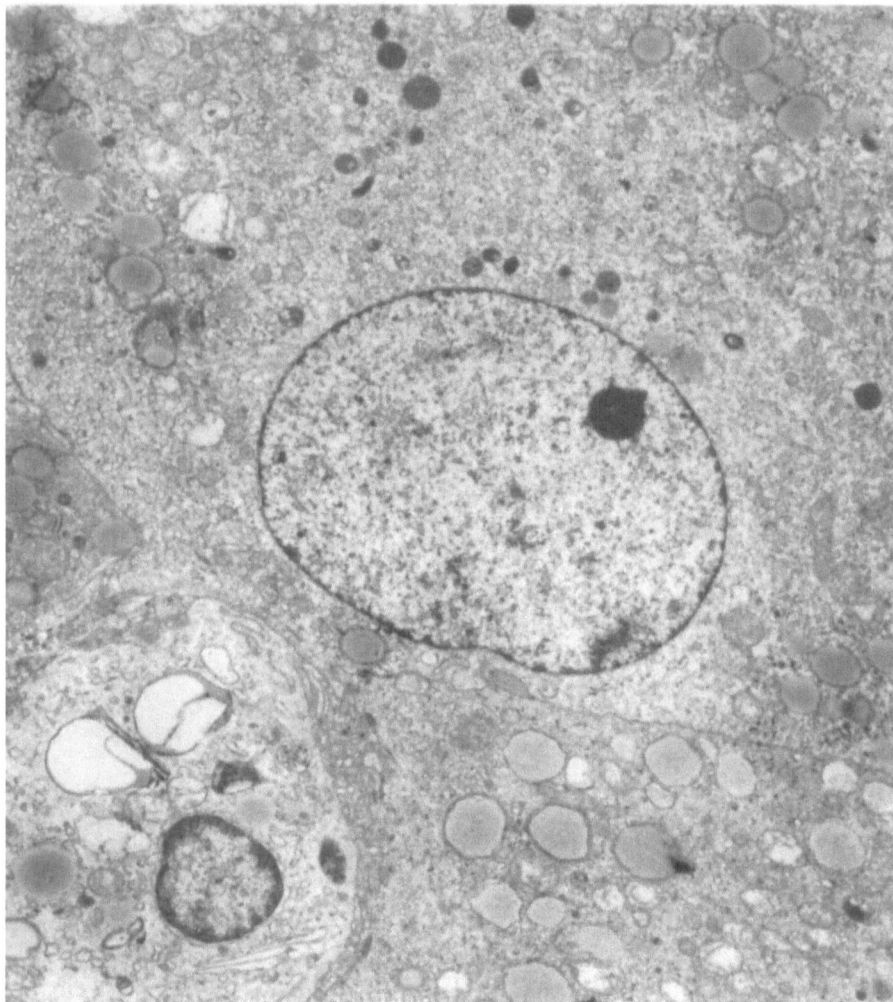

Fig. 7. Functioning and degenerating luteal cells of a Corpus luteum cyst showing abundance of smooth endoplasmic vesicles and lipid droplets. × 7900

The lining epithelium is composed of flat, cuboidal or columnar cells, and resembles endometrial or endosalpingeal epithelium (Fig. 9). Inclusion cysts formerly believed to be present only in the ovaries of peri- and postmenopausal women, resulting from repeated ovulation with trapping of surface epithelium in the cortex, also occur in fetal ovaries and in ovaries of infants, adolescents, and young women (BLAUSTEIN et al. 1982). From both light- and electron microscopic observations it can be concluded that ovarian inclusion cysts are hormonally induced. Ultrastructurally, the lining cells are similar to peritoneal mesothelial cells, but show higher grades of cytoplasmic organization, their cytoplasm containing lysosomes, lipids and secreting vacuoles, and their apical membranes carrying abundant microvilli and cilia.

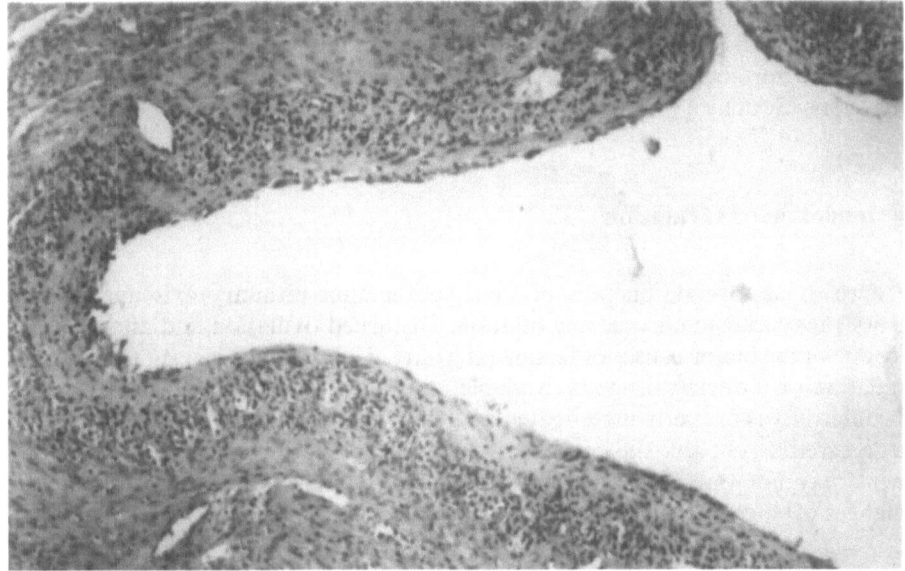

Fig. 8. Theca lutein cyst with hyperplastic theca layer and complete degeneration of granulosa

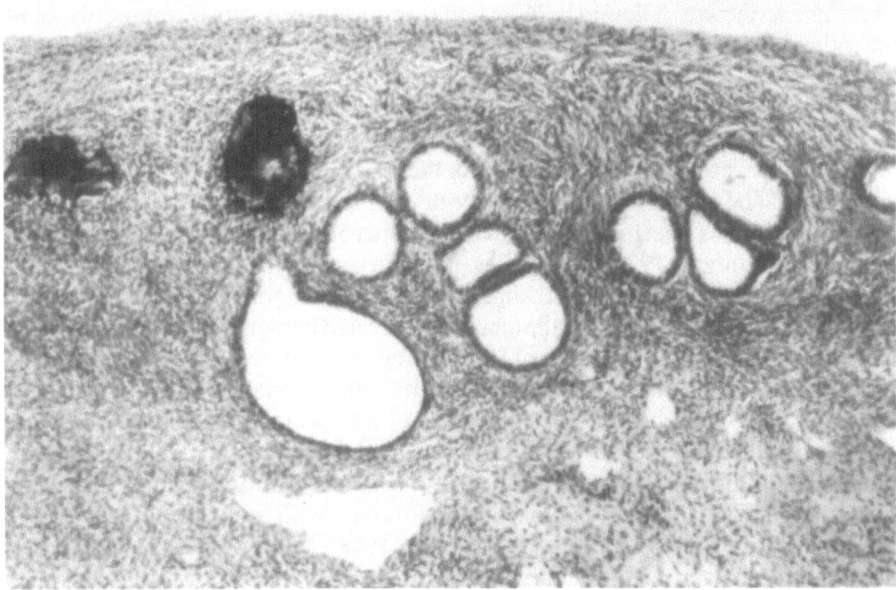

Fig. 9. Cortical inclusion cysts and calcium deposits in postmenopausal ovary

The hormonal responsiveness of cells lining inclusion cysts was further demonstrated by an ARIAS STELLA-like phenomenon in women who had ectopic pregnancy. Metaplastic alterations have been found in menarchal and perimenopausal ovaries, but were not seen in inclusion cysts of premenarchal ovaries.

Common epithelial tumours of the ovary, benign, borderline, and malignant, are believed to be derived from the multipotential coelomic epithelium that covers the surface of the ovary and lines invaginations and cystic epithelial inclusions (Scully 1979).

8 Induction of Ovulation

Failure or abnormal function of the hypothalamic-pituitary axis and/or the ovaries may lead to chronic anovulation. Disturbed ovulation and anovulation are one of the major causes of female infertility. Today a wide range of ovulation initiating or inducing drugs is available and extensively used. If the cause for the infertility is properly investigated and the type and dosage of the appropriate drug carefully chosen, the results can be excellent; however, inadequate treatment may not only cause severe side-effects, but also induce morphological changes of the ovaries simulating neoplastic lesions.

8.1 Antioestrogens

Clomiphene citrate (Clomid: CC) is the antioestrogen most commonly used for induction of ovulation. Clomiphene, a nonsteroidal compound structurally related to diethylstilbestrol, is a mixture of two isomeres: cis and trans. It is but one member of a large family of antioestrogenic acting triphenylethylene derivatives, some of them widely used in basic research, others – such as tamoxifen – have proven to be effective drugs in the treatment of hormonally responsive neoplasms. The antioestrogenic activity of clomiphene and other triphenylethylene derivatives has been demonstrated by numerous investigators (Lunan-Burnett and Klopper 1975). Acting as an antioestrogen, clomiphene has been shown to attenuate vaginal epithelial maturation, antagonize several oestrogen-dependent properties of cervical mucus, and reverse benign and malignant endometrial changes. Administration of clomiphene to untreated or oestrogen-treated postmenopausal women results in progressive endometrial atrophy.

The mode of action and the sequence of events in clomiphene induced ovulation is not fully understood. According to current concepts, the ability of clomiphene to initiate an ovulatory sequence is primarily, and perhaps exclusively, due to its ability to be recognized and interact with oestrogen receptors at the level of the hypothalamus (Kato et al. 1968; Wentz et al. 1976). Acting as an antioestrogen, clomiphene is thought to displace endogenous oestrogen from hypothalamic oestrogen receptor sites. The decrease in intracellular receptor concentration in the hypothalamus initiates an hypooestrogenic state and induces the synthesis and release of LH-RH to stimulate the secretion of pituitary FSH and LH, thus initiating the sequence of events that result in a normal cycle. Follicular development once initiated, however, results in increased concentrations of estradiol, two or five times greater than during spontaneous cycles (Vandenberg and Yen 1973). Midcycle LH-peak, also up to five times higher than during normal cycles, occurs in response to the increased estradiol levels, on average 12 to 15 days after the first day of treatment, resulting in ovulation and development of corpus luteum which is characterized by a progesterone output higher than in spontaneous cycles.

The overall fertility effect of clomiphene may not only reflect the interactions with the hypothalamus, but also with other levels of the hypothalamic-pituitary-ovarian axis (ADASHI 1984).

Both the ovulation inducing effect and the pregnancy rate can be significantly improved by combining clomiphene with HCG, obviously due to enhancement of the LH surge. Essentially, all patients who have failed to ovulate on CC but who have evidence of oestrogenic response (cervical mucus changes, high serum estradiol levels), are good candidates for combined CC and HCG treatment. Hyperprolactinemia may be a cause of CC resistant anovulation, however, there is some evidence that in such cases the combination with prolactin-inhibiting drugs such as bromocryptine may enhance CC treatment and restore positive feed-back mechanism and ovulation.

Due to relatively low side effects CC is regarded as the drug of the first choice in anovulatory infertility but the patients must be carefully selected. The overall pregnancy rate following CC administration is 30 to 40% when large series are considered. Multiple pregnancy (mainly twins) have been reported to occur in 2 to 12% and reflect the occurence of multiple ovulation.

8.2 Human Gonadotropins

The first attempt to induce ovulation with a human pituitary gonadotropin preparation was reported by GEMZELL et al. (1958, 1965, 1970) however, the availability of human gonadotropins obtained by extracting pituitary glands from autopsy specimens was very limited and the side effects severe. Since then, both the gonadotropin preparations and treatment schemes have been standardized greatly reducing toxicity (INSLER et al. 1968; RABAU et al. 1967; BETTENDORF and INSLER 1970). Human gonadotropins are now widely available commercially and are extracted from the urine of menopausal women (HMG). Gonadotropin treatment is indicated in patients who fail to respond to CC (and HCG) treatment. It is the method of choice for induction of ovulation in amenorrhoeic women with normal prolactin and low oestrogen.

As HMG and HCG treatment may not only cause severe side effects but also carries a higher risk of ovarian overstimulation compared to CC therapy, patients must be both carefully selected and continually monitored. The effective dose for each individual is determined by initiating treatment with a low dose of HMG and increasing it in a stepwise fashion, correlating it with the daily values of plasma or urinary oestrogen levels, when these indicate the presence of a mature follicle, HCG is administered in a single dose, usually of 10000 IU, 24 or 48 hours following the last HMG injection. Individual variations in response often occur and may cause either under- or over-stimulation of the ovaries. Severe ovarian hyperstimulation syndrome – ovarian enlargement greater than 10 cm, ascites and hydrothorax – has been reported in 1–3% of cases but should be completely preventable with continuous oestrogen measurement and sonographic monitoring. If it does occur, the symptoms usually disappear within a few weeks after treatment withdrawal; however, if the patient has become pregnant, placental HCG prevents prompt resolution and indeed may exacerbate the cystic enlargement. Such cases obviously require intensive follow-up.

8.3 Gonadotropin-Releasing Hormone (Gn-RH)

Gonadotropin-releasing hormone in its synthetic form is a new effective drug for inducing ovulation in patients with endogenous Gn-RH deficiency. Administration by a single (bolus) injection following CC administration has been effective in causing a surge of LH and ovulation of approximately 50% of previous CC resistent patients. The development of a computer-controlled portable injection pump (Zyclomat) now enables an uninterrupted pulsatile intravenous self administration of GnRH which in adequate dosage and sequence induces monovulation in nearly 100%.

8.4 Ovarian Hyperstimulation Syndrome

Ovarian hyperstimulation is a recognized complication of gonadotropic therapy for induction of ovulation. It has been classified as mild, moderate, and severe. Patient monitoring with ultrasound reveals mild hyperstimulation in up to 44% of cases of effective gonadotropin treatment (McArdle et al. 1983). It is characterized by a non-symptomatic multifollicular cystic ovarian enlargement between 5 to 7 cm, reaching a maximum 5 to 10 days after completion of treatment. Patients with a prior history of functional ovarian cysts or polycystic ovarian disease are at a greater risk of hyperstimulation (Kistner 1966). In moderate hyperstimulation ovarian enlargement does not exceed 10 cm. The severe form of hyperstimulation syndrome (Rabau et al. 1967) consists of the development of large multilocular cysts with ascites, with or without hydrothorax and may also be associated with haemoconcentration and coagulation abnormalities. Haemorrhage into the cysts is common, torsion and rupture may occur leading to symptoms of acute abdomen. This form of extreme hyperstimulation is seen mainly after HCG and HMG therapy for ovulation induction. Only few cases have been described after clomiphene induced ovulations (Schenker and Weinstein 1978; Holtz et al. 1982; Chow and Choo 1984). Microscopically, the cysts are lined by a thin layer of luteinized granulosa cells, which is separated by a small strip of collagenous tissue from an external layer of luteinized theca cells (Fig. 10). There is marked oedema of both the luteinized theca layer and the ovarian stroma which may contain islands and strands of luteinized interstitial cells. Patients with moderate or severe OHSS should be hospitalized and carefully controlled by urinary oestrogen measurements and ultrasonographic monitoring of the ovaries. There is no indication for aspiration of ovarian cysts nor surgical intervention unless torsion or rupture with intraabdominal

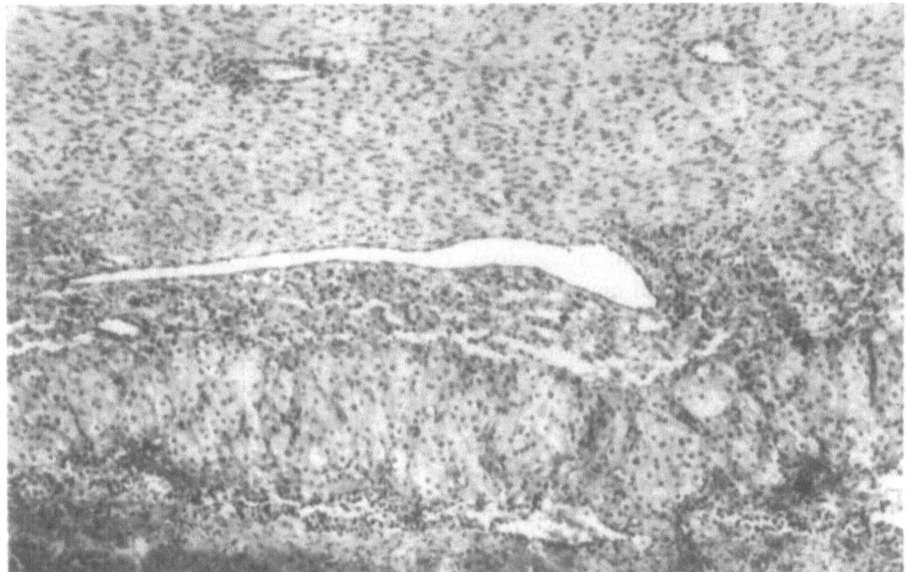

Fig. 10. Theca lutein cyst from ovarian hyperstimulation syndrome

bleeding occurs. The recognition of ovarian enlargement as a non-neoplastic hormonally induced lesion is of great importance to avoid unnecessarily extensive surgical treatment.

9 Hyperplastic Lesions

9.1 Stromal Hyperplasia and Hyperthecosis

A common feature found in postmenopausal ovaries is the predominance of the stromal pattern, partly due to active proliferation of stromal cells, which may possess varying degrees of hormonal activity, and to the regression of follicles, corpora albicantia and medullary connective tissue. In the postmenopausal ovary, the stroma consists of undifferentiated mesenchymal cells which are inert to gonadotropic stimulation, and gonadotropin-sensitive steroid-producing interstitial cells, which account for approximately one third of the entire stromal compartment. Steroid-producing interstitial cells show accumulation of plasma lipids and high activities of oxido reductases (enzymatically active stroma cells: EASC) (WOODRUFF et al. 1963; SCULLY and COHEN 1964; PFLEIDERER and TEUFEL 1968; JANOVSKI and PARAMANANDHAN 1973). Ultramicroscopically, they reveal an assortment of cytoplasmic organelles characteristic of steroid-producing cells similar to those of theca and lutein cells. As suggested from incubation studies, the enzymatically active interstitial cells of the postmenopausal ovary are a main source of androgens and responsible for the changing pattern of ovarian steroidogenesis after the menopause. There is no clear border between normal proliferation of stromal cells in the postmenopausal ovary and non-neoplastic stromal hyperplasia. The term "stromal hyperthecosis" refers specifically to the presence of steroid-active (luteinized) interstitial cells in a stroma that is usually hyperplastic. Although more common in older women, both processes may be encountered during reproductive years and in some cases may be associated with androgenic manifestations. Non-neoplastic stromal hyperplasia occurs bilaterally, which is an important criteria when making the differential diagnosis with the various types of solid mesenchymal ovarian tumours which in general develop unilaterally. Microscopically, stromal hyperplasia and hyperthecosis usually involve the medulla of the ovary but may also overgrow the cortex in a diffuse or nodular pattern. In extreme cases, nearly all of the parenchyma is replaced by multinodular or diffuse masses of stroma. The proliferating cells resemble normal stromal cells, but appear slightly hyperplastic. Lipid stains may reveal intracytoplasmic lipid droplets in varying amounts and focal distribution.

YOUNG and SCULLY (1984) recently described a special form of stromal hyperplasia denominated ovarian fibromatosis in young women, some who had been investigated for menstrual abnormalities or symptoms suggestive of excess androgen production. On gross examination the enlarged ovaries were firm and white and included small cystic cavitations. Microscopically, a diffuse proliferation of fibroblasts was found, frequently with the production of abundant collagen surrounding residual ovarian structures. In one of the cases reported, lutein cells were identified in the fibromatous areas and in another case they were found in the adjacent ovarian stroma. The androgenic manifestations correlated with the presence of lutein cells, either within the lesions or the adjacent ovarian stroma.

Similar to polycystic ovaries, stromal hyperplasia and hyperthecosis can also induce endometrial hyperplasia and carcinoma. There is rising evidence, however, that these "oestrogenic" phenomena in fact are the result of peripheral conversion of androgens produced by the ovarian stromal cells to oestrogens (estrone).

9.2 Luteal Hyperplasia and Pregnancy Luteoma

Pregnancy luteomas are single or multinodular tumour-like hyperplasias of lutein cells that develop during normal or abnormal pregnancy and regress spontaneously during the puerperium. HCG has been implicated as an obligate factor in the pathogenesis of the luteomas, but this hormone is possibly not the sole aetiological factor and no relationship between tumour development and hormone concentration has been found. The nodules are in general discovered as incidental findings on occasion of Cesarean section or surgical procedures for other indications during pregnancy (STERNBERG and BARCLAY 1966).

On gross examination the tumours are soft, well-circumscribed yellow-brown or brown nodules measuring up to 20 cm in diameter. They may contain areas of haemorrhage or small cystic inclusions. The single or multiple nodules appear

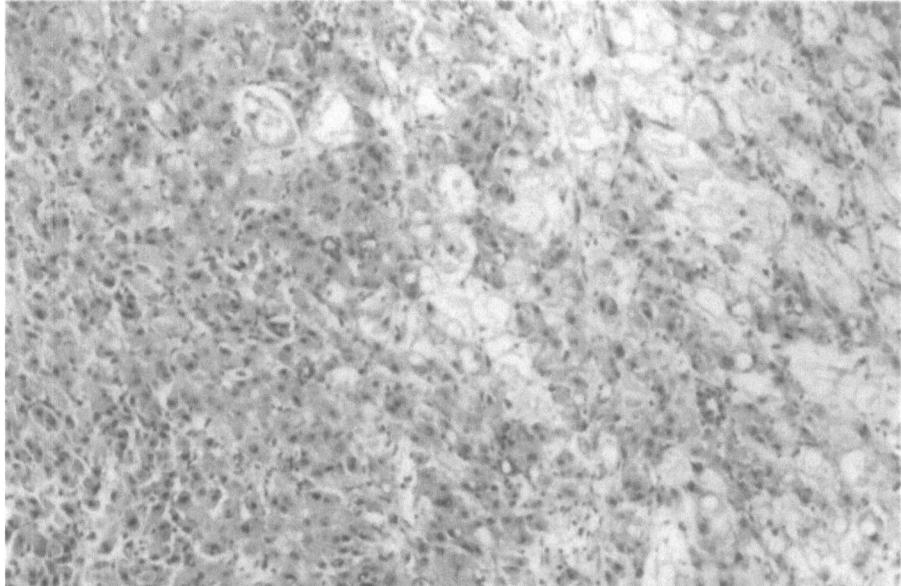

Fig. 11. Pregnancy luteoma

mostly unilateral, but the frequency of bilaterality is difficult to determine because lesions of microscopic size may be present in a grossly normal, contralateral ovary. Microscopically the nodules are composed of large round or polygonal cells. The cytoplasm is abundant and eosinophilic, sometimes finely granular or vacuolated. The cells form compact solid or vacuolated complexes, occasionally they are arranged in cords, or lining small glandular-like spaces (Fig. 11). Within the intra- and extracellular vacuoles, PAS-positive colloid droplets of varying size similar to those found in the corpus luteum of pregnancy are seen.

Slight or moderate nuclear polymorphism, multinucleation and mitoses may simulate malignant atypia giving rise to misinterpretation. Involuting luteomas are characterized by degenerative cytological changes such as nuclear pyknosis, swelling and vacuolization (ballooning) of the cytoplasm and ingrowth of connective tissue.

Ultramicroscopical examination reveals an assortment of cytoplasmic constituents that is typical of steroid-hormone producing cells i.e. abundant vesicular smooth endoplasmic reticulum, mitochondria of tubular type, and lipid droplets (Fig. 12). In approximately a quarter of the cases reported in the literature hirsutism of different degrees has been observed (NORRIS and TAYLOR 1967).

9.3 Hilus Cell Hyperplasia

Hilar cells are found in islands or strands mostly in juxtaposition to non-medullated nerve fibers and blood vessels of the ovarian hilus. These cells are round

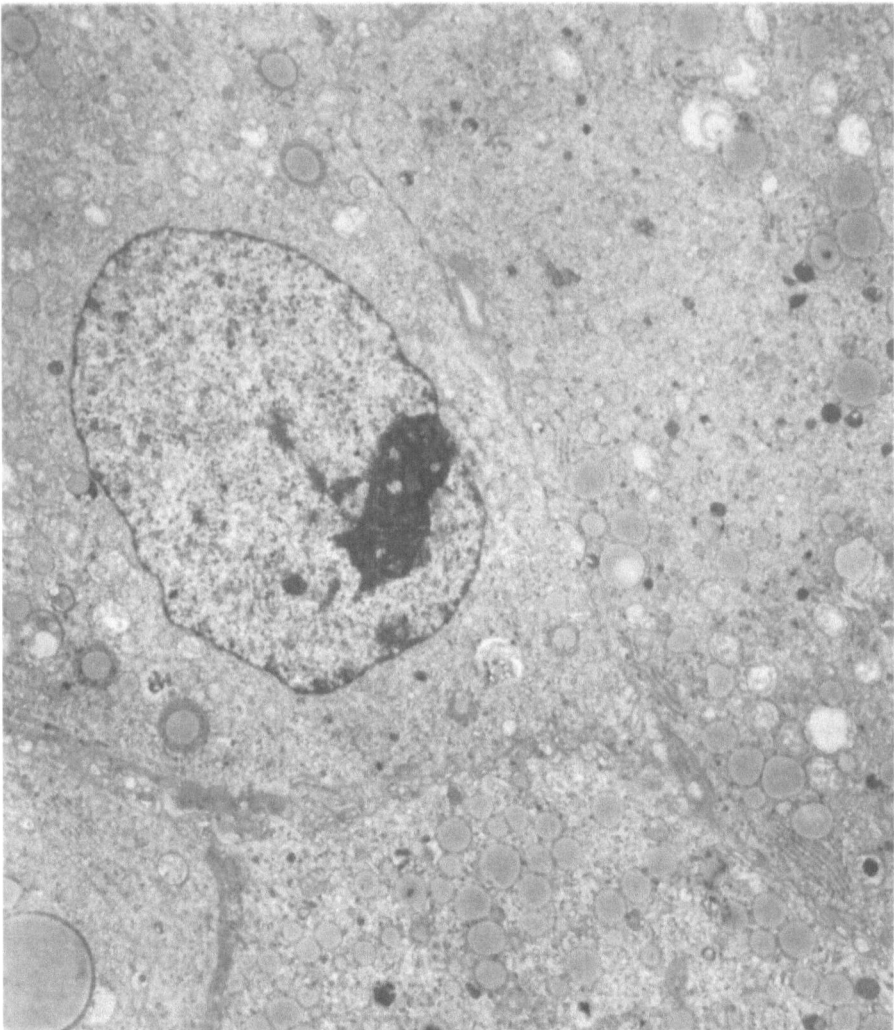

Fig. 12. Electron microscopical structure of lutein cells of pregnancy luteoma

or oval, have well defined round nuclei and abundant eosinophilic cytoplasm of foamy and finely granular appearence. Like their counterparts in the testis – the Leydig cells – they may contain crystalloids of Reinke and lipochrome pigment.

Hilar cells are most prominent at birth, puberty, pregnancy, menopause and in patients with choriocarcinoma. Sternberg et al. (1953) has shown that the response of hilar cells to human chorionic gonadotropin (HCG) stimulation is similar to that observed with Leydig cells of the testis. In postmenopausal ovaries, hilar cells may show marked nuclear polymorphism, the cell nests being intermingled with dense collagenous tissue.

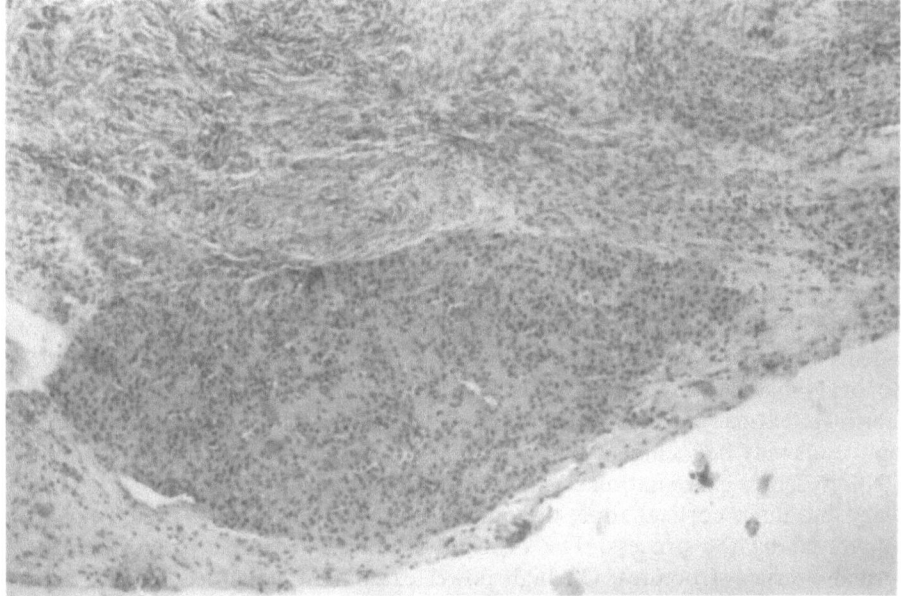

Fig. 13. Hilus cell hyperplasia of post menopausal ovary

Hilus cell hyperplasia, unless obstrusive, may be difficult to recognize by routine examination of the ovaries because of the focal distribution of hilar cell nests and a considerable individual variability (Fig. 13). In ovaries of non-pregnant women of reproductive age hilus cell hyperplasia may be found in association with diffuse stromal hyperplasia or hyperthecosis. There is no clear border between nodular hyperplasia of hilar cells and hilus cell tumours of the ovary, nor are there significant cytomorphological differences between the cell constituents of both lesions. As proven by enzyme- and immunohistochemical studies hilar (LEYDIG) cells are preferred sites of androgen biosynthesis in both normal and pathological conditions (KURMAN et al. 1978). Many of the patients affected with diffuse or nodular hilus cell hyperplasia develop clinical signs and symptoms of hyperandrogenism, but also hyperoestrogenic manifestation such as glandular and adenomatous endometrial hyperplasia have been reported.

10 Massive Oedema of the Ovary

Massive oedema of the ovary is defined by the WHO as a tumour-like condition in which there is marked enlargement of one or both ovaries due to extreme accumulation of oedema fluid in the ovarian stroma. The lesion was firstly described by KALSTONE et al. (1970). The authors postulated that massive oedema was caused by lymphatic obstruction due to recurrent torsion of an otherwise normal ovary but in 1971 SCULLY suggested that at least some cases might result from a primary hyperproliferation of the stroma followed by secondary oedema.

Massive oedema is predominantly found in young women, the average age of the patients being 21 years with a range of 6 to 33 years (NASSAR et al. 1976, CHERVENAK et al. 1980, YOUNG and SCULLY 1984). The most common presenting symptoms are abdominal pain and abdominal swelling. In some cases the sudden onset of pain may mimic acute abdomen. Menstrual irregularities or symptoms suggesting excess androgen production may precede the acute symptoms. Massive oedema is usually unilateral. Partial or complete torsion was noted in nearly 50% of the cases. The size of the ovary involved by massive oedema ranged from 5.5 to 35 cm. In a case reported by NASSAR et al. (1976) the ovary had a weight of 2400 g. On gross inspection, the enlarged ovary had a white, opaque surface. The sectioned surfaces had a watery appearence, small cysts may be included.

Microscopic examination shows loose oedematous tissue occupying the medullary and inner cortical zone, the outer cortex forming a small pseudocapsule uninvolved by the process. The oedematous parenchyma surrounds residual normal ovarian structures. On high power examination the oedematous areas show spindle-shaped cells widely separated by interstitial pale staining fluid. Focal necrosis or haemorrhage may be present. Vessels and lymphatics appear prominent due to extreme dilatation. In addition to oedema, aggregates of lutein cells and foci of fibromatosis have been described.

The histogenesis of massive oedema still causes much controversy. According to SCULLY (1971) massive oedema is secondary to a primary diffuse hyperplasia of the ovarian stroma or thecal cells possibly due to torsion of an abnormal, already enlarged organ. Luteinization in cases of massive oedema may also be explained on the basis of preexistent stromal hyperthecosis. In some cases androgenic manifestations (hirsutism or virilism) were correlated with the presence of luteinization accompanying oedematous transformation (ROTH 1971; VASQUEZ et al. 1982). On gross examination massive oedema may be confused with any ovarian tumour characterized by prominent oedema such as fibromas, thecomas or KRUKENBERG tumours.

Wedge resection is adequate in most cases of massive oedema of the ovary but unfortunately in most cases it may not be possible to differentiate massive oedema from a true neoplasia by gross evaluation at the time of operation (KLEINER et al. 1978). In such cases a conservative surgical approach is advisable (excision of the only involved or larger of two involved ovaries) and the decision for more radical treatment postponed until a final diagnosis is made on paraffin embedded tissue.

11 Endometriosis

Ovarian endometriosis accounts for 80% of all pelvic endometriosis. Non-neoplastic endometriosis may range from small microscopic foci to large so-called chocolate cysts. On microscopic examination fresh implants of functioning endometrium are found predominantly within the cortical region of the ovaries or may be located at the surface of the ovary. The presence of endometrial type stroma associated with endometrial type glands is a precondition for the diagnosis of endometriosis which should be distinguished from inclusion cysts of the surface epithelium and from endometrial-like cysts that are lined by epithelium resembling that of the fallopian tube (endosalpingiosis). In functioning implants the ectopic endometrium responds to hormonal cyclicity but the estrogen and progesterone-induced morphologic changes are less pronounced than in the uterine mucosa. As demonstrated by immunohistochemical technique oestrogen receptor localization is similar to that of eutopic endometrium but of higher variability than in cyclic endometrium (BUR et al. 1987). Pregnancy and progestational agents can induce a marked decidual response of the stromal components. Endometriotic cysts may be single, but are more frequently multiple. They tend to increase in size with the periodical bleeding that occurs during menstrual cycle, in severe cases resulting in adhesive conglomerate tumours of the adnexa. An unequivocal diagnosis of endometriotic cysts can only be made if both endometrial type glands and stroma are present, but this is not always the case. One or both of these elements can be found completely obliterated by repeated bleeding and consequent pressure atrophy leaving a thick-walled fibrotic cyst in which the fibroblastic and collagenized stroma contains haemosiderin laden macrophages (pseudoxanthoma cells). Ovarian endometriosis may give rise to endometrioid type carcinoma (FERREIRA and CLAYTON 1958; DOCKERTY 1962; RIDLEY 1966; CZERNOBILSKY et al. 1970). Since endometrioid carcinoma is a common type of primary ovarian cancer it may be difficult to determine what percentage of endometrioid carcinomas of the ovary arise from preexistent ectopic endometrium unless both lesions are found combined or in direct continuity with normal appearing ectopic endometrium as atypical hyperplastic or frankly malignant endometrium. Nuclear and cellular atypia due to degenerative processes of the epithelium lining endometrioid cysts may occasionally mimic premalignant change (CZERNOBILSKY and MORRIS 1979).

12 Ectopic Decidua

Owing to their histogenetic origin from the steroid-sensitive subcoelomic mesenchyme the ovarian stromal cells may undergo decidual transformation during pregnancy, in association with hormone producing trophoblastic and other tumours, or by various conditions with high circulating levels of oestrogen and progesterone. Pseudodecidual reaction – similar in microscopic appearance to true decidua – may be found in non-pregnant and postmenopausal women secondary to pelvic inflammation (histamine reaction?) or without any apparent cause. The most frequent site of focal decidualization is the submesothelial stromal layer. Sometimes, the decidual nests form small polypoid protrusions on the ovarian surface. Histologically, ectopic decidual cells are undistinguishable from their counterparts seen in the endometrium, being characterized by abundant pale basophilic cytoplasm, clearly defined cell borders and round nuclei with distinct nucleoli. Lymphocyte infiltration and rich vascularity are common features of ectopic decidual nests.

References

Adashi FY, Rock JA, Guzick D, Wentz AC, Jones GS, Jones HW (1981) Fertility following bilateral ovarian wedge resection: a critical analysis of 90 consecutive cases of the polycystic ovary syndrom. Fertil Steril 56:320–325

Adashi EY (1984) Clomiphene citrate: Mechanism (s) and site (s) of action – a hypothesis revisited. Fertil Steril 42:331–344

Barakat BY, Ances IF, Tang CK, Fajer AB (1979) 46,XY gonadal dysgenesis with secondary amenorrhea, virilization, and bilateral gonadoblastoms. South Med J 72:1163–1165

Bettendorf G, Insler V (1970) Clinical application of human gonadotropins (eds) G. Thieme, Stuttgart

Blaustein A, Kantius M, Kaganowicz A, Pervez N, Wells J (1982) Inclusions in ovaries of females aged 1–30 years. Int J Gynecol Pathol 1:145–154

Bonakdar MI, Peisner DB (1980) Gonadoblastoma with a 45,X karyotype Obstet Gynecol 56:748–750

Bur ME, Greene GL, Press MF (1987) Estrogen receptor localization in formalin-fixed, paraffin-embedded endometrium and endometriotic tissues. Int J Gynecol Pathol 6:140–151

Campenhout J van, Vauclair R, Maraghi K (1972) Gonadotropin-resistant ovaries in primary amenorrhea. Obstet Gynecol 40:6–12

Channing CP, Anderson LD, Hoover DJ, Kolena J, Osteen KG, Pomerantz SH Tanabe K (1982) The role of nonsteroidal regulators in control of oocyte and follicular maturation. Recent Progr Horm Res 38:331–408

Chervenak FA, Castadot MJ, Wiedermann J, Sedlis A (1980) Massive ovarian edema: review of world literature and report of two cases. Obstet Gynecol Surv 35:677–684

Chow KK, Choo HT (1984) Ovarian hyperstimulation syndrome with clomiphenecitrate. Case report. Brit J Obstet Gynaecol 91:1051–1052

Clement PB, Scully RE (1979) Large solitary luteinized follicle cyst of pregnancy and puerperium. A clinico-pathological analysis of 8 cases. Am J Surg Pathol 4:431–438

Cohen MB (1979) Surgical management of infertility in the polycystic ovary syndrome. In: Givens JR (ed) The infertile female. Yearbook Med Publ Chicago

Coulam CB, Gallenberg MM, Webb MJ, Gaffey TA (1982) The absence of H-Y antigen in XY gonads grossly resembling ovaries. Am J Obstet Gynecol 142:925

Curtis WR, White BJ, Lucky AW, Roche-Bender N, Knab DR, Johansonbaugh RE (1980) Gonadal dysgenesis with mosaicism and a non-fluorescent Y chromosome: Report of two cases with correlation of clinical pathologic, and cytogenetic findings. Am J Obstet Gynecol 136:639–645

Czernobilsky B, Silverman BB, Mikuta JJ (1970) Endometrioid carcinoma of the ovary. A clinicopathologic study of 75 cases. Cancer 26:1141–1152

Czernobilsky B, Morris WJ (1979) A histologic study of ovarian endometriosis with emphasis on hyperplastic and atypical changes. Obstet Gynecol 53:318–328

Damjanov I, Klauber G (1980) Microscopic gonadoblastoma in dysgenetic gonad of an infant: an ultrastructural study. Urology 15:605–609

Dewhurst CJ, DeKoss EB, Ferreira HP (1975) The resistent ovary syndrome. Brit J Obst Gynecol 82:341–345

Dignam WJ, Pion RJ, Lamb EJ (1964) Plasma androgens in women. II. Patients with polycystic ovaries and hirsutism. Acta Endocrinol (Kbh) 45:254–271

DiZerega GS, Goebelsmann U, Nakamura R (1982) Identification of protein (s) secreted by the preovulatory ovary which suppresses the follicle response to gonadotropins. J Clin Endocrinol Metabolism 54:1091–1096

Dockerty MB (1962) Malignancy complicating endometriosis. Am J Obstet Gynecol 83:175–179

Erickson GF, Hsueh AJW, Quigley ME, Rebar RW, Yen SSC (1979) Functional studies of aromatase activity in human granulosa cells from normal and polycystic ovaries. J Clin Endocr Metab 49:514–519

Ferreira HP, Clayton SG (1958) Three cases of malignant changes in endometriosis including two cases arising in rectovaginal septum. J Obstet Gynecol Br Emp 65:41–44

Gemzell C, Disczfalusy E, Tillinger KG (1958) Clinical effect of human pituitary follicle stimulating hormone (FSH). J Clin Endocrinol 18:1333–1348

Gemzell C (1965) Induction of ovulation with human gonadotrophins. Recent Progr Horm Res 21:179–204

Gemzell C (1970) Experiences with human pituitary gonadotrophins in infertile women. In: Butler JK (ed) Development in the Pharmacology and Clinical Uses of Human Gonadotrophins. SD Searle & Co. High Wycombe, England

Goldzieher JW, Axelrod LR (1963) Clinical and biochemical features of polycystic ovarian disease. Fertil Steril 14:631–641

Gunnala S, Eskin BA, Bartuska DG (1981) Pure gonadal dysgenesis with microscopic ovarian streak and gonadoblastoma. Obstet Gynecol 57:58–61

Hall JL, Wachtel SS (1980) Primary sex determination: genetics and biochemistry. Mol Cell Biochem 33:49–66

Haseltine FP, Ohno S (1981) Mechanisms of gonadal differentiation. Science 211:1272–1278

Hjörtrup A, Kehler H, Lockwood K, Hasner E (1983) Long term clinical effects of ovarian wedge resection in polycystic ovarian syndrome. Acta Obstet Cynecol Scand 62:55–57

Holtz G, Kling OR, Miller DD, Wilson DA (1982) Ovarian hyperstimulation syndrome caused by clomiphene citrate. South Med J 75:368–370

Insler V, Melmed H, Mshiah S, Monselise M, Lunenfeld B, Rabau E (1968) Functional classification of patients selected for gonadotropic therapy. Obstet Gynecol 32:620–626

Irvine WJ, Chan MM, Scarth L et al. (1968) Immunological aspects of premature ovarian failure associated with idiopathic Addison's disease. Lancet 2:883–887

Irvine WJ, Chan MMW, Scarth C (1969) The further characterization of autoantibodies reactive with extra-adrenal steroid-producing cells in patients with adrenal disorders. Clin Exp Immunol 4:489–503

Ito T, Horton R (1971) The source of plasma dihydrotestosterone in man. J Clin Invest Metab 50:1621–1627

Janovski NA, Paramanandhan TL (1973) Ovarian tumors. Tumor and tumor-like conditions of the ovaries, fallopian tubes and ligaments of the uterus. G. Thieme, Stuttgart

Kalstone CE, Jaffe RB, Abell MR (1970) Massive edema of the ovary simulating fibroma. Obstet Gynecol 34:564–571

Kato J, Kobayashi F, Villec CA (1968) Effect of clomiphene on the uptake of estradiol by the anterior hypothalamus und hypophysis. Endocrinol 82:1049–1052

Kinch RAH, Plunket ER, Smout MS, Carl DH (1965) Primary ovarian failure. Amer J Obstet Gynecol 91:630–644

Kim MH (1974) "Gonadotropin-resistent ovaries" syndrome in association with secondary amenorrhea. Am J Obstet Gynecol 120:257–263

King CR, Magensis E, Bennett S (1979) Pregnancy and the Turner Syndrome. Obstet Gynecol 52:617–624

Kirschner MA, Jacobs J (1971) Combined ovarian and abdominal vein catheterization to determine site (s) of androgen overproduction in hirsute women. J Clin Endocrinol Metab 33:199–209

Kistner RW (1966) Use of clomiphene citrate, human chorionic gonadotropin, and human menopausal gonadotropin for induction of ovulation in the human female. Fertil Steril 17:569–583

Kleiner GK, Solomon L, Greston WM, Lev-Gur M (1978) Wedge resection in massive edema of the ovary. Am J Obstet Gynecol 137:107

Koninckx PR (1981) New aspects of ovarian function in man and in rat. Thesis, Katholieke Universiteit Leuven, Fakulteit Geneeskunde, Belgium

Kurman RJ, Andrade D, Goebelsmann U, Taylor CR (1978) An immunohistological study of steroid localization in Sertoli-Leydig tumors of the ovary and testis. Cancer (Philad) 42:1772–1783

Kurman RJ, Goebelsmann U, Taylor CR, Bchir MD (1981) Localization of steroid hormones in functional ovarian tumors. In: DeLellis RA: Diagnostic Immunohistochemistry. Masson, Paris

Kurman RJ, Ganjei P, Nadji M (1984) Contributions of immunocytochemistry to the diagnosis and study of ovarian neoplasms. Int J Gynecol Pathol 3:3–26

Lintern-Moore S, Peters H, Moore GPM, Faber M (1974) Follicular development in the infant human ovary. J Reprod Fert 39:53–64

Lunan-Burnett C, Klopper A (1975) Antiestrogens: A review. Clin Endocr 4:551–572

Luzzatto R, Murray JM, Gallager HS (1979) Gonadoblastoma associated with malignant teratoma. South Med J 72:624–627

Mahesh VB, Greenblatt RB (1964) Steroid secretions in the normal and polycystic ovary. Recent Progr Horm Res 20:341–394

McArdle CR, Seibel M, Weinstein F, Hann LE, Nickerson C, Taymor ML (1983) Induction of ovulation monitored by ultrasound. Radiology 148:809–812

Moltz L, Schwartz U, Pickartz H, Hammerstein J, Wolf U (1981) XY gonadal dysgenesis: aberrant testicular differentiation in the presence of H-Y antigen. Obstet Gynecol 58:17–25

Moraes-Ruehsen M, Blizzard RM, Garcia-Bunuel R, Jones GS (1972) Autoimmunity and ovarian failure. Am J Obstet Gynecol 112:693–703

Nassar TR, Virgilio LA, Abdul-Karim RW (1976) Massive edema of the ovary. A case report and a review of the literature. Obstet Gynecol 47:775–805

Norris HJ, Taylor JB (1967) Nodular theca lutein hyperplasia of pregnancy (so-called "pregnancy luteoma"). A clinical and pathologic study of 15 cases. Am J Clin Pathol 47:557–566

Peters H (1980) The Ovary. Paul Elek (ed) Granada. London

Pfleiderer A, Teufel G (1968) Incidence and histochemical investigation of enzymatically active cells in stroma of ovarian tumors. Am J Obstet Gynecol 102:997

Pickartz H, Moltz L, Altenähr E (1980) XY (H-Y) Gonadal Dysgenesis. Virchows Arch path Anat 389:103–112

Rabau E, Serr DM, Mashiah S, Insler V, Salomy M, Lunenfeld B (1967) Current concepts in the treatment of anovulation. Br Med J 4:446–449

Rebar RW (1983) The reproductive age: chronic anovulation. In: Serra GB (ed) The Ovary. Raven Press, New York

Rebar RW, Rebar MF, Silva De SA (1983) The reproductive age: premature ovarian failure. In: Serra GB (ed) The ovary. Raven Press, New York

Ridley JH (1966) Primary adenocarcinoma in implant of endometriosis. Obstet Gynecol 77:261–267

Robboy STJ, Miller TH, Donahoe PK, Jahre C, Welch WR, Haseltine FP, Miller WA, Atkins L, Crawford JD (1982) Dysgenesis of testicular and streak gonads in the syndrome of mixed gonadal dysgenesis. Perspective derived from a clinicopathologic analysis of twenty-one cases. Hum Pathol 13:700–716

Roth LM (1971) Massive ovarian edema with stroma luteinization: a nearly recognized virilizing syndrome apparently related to partial torsion of the mesovarium. Am J Clin Path 55:757–760

Scully RE (1953) Gonadoblastom. A gonadal tumor related to dysgerminoma (seminoma) and capable of sex hormone production. Cancer 6:455–681

Scully RE (1970) Gonadoblastoma, a review of 74 cases. Cancer 25:1340–1356

Scully RE (1971) Case records of the Massachusetts General Hospital (case 24 – 1971). N Engl J Med 284:1369–1375

Scully RE (1979) Atlas of tumor pathology. Second series, Fasc 16. Tumors of the ovary and maldeveloped gonads. Armed Forces Inst. of Pathol Washington D.C.

Scully RE, Cohen RB (1964) Oxidative-enzyme activities in normal and pathologic human ovaries. Obstet Gynecol 24:667

Singh RP, Carr DH (1966) The anatomy and histology of XO human embryos and fetuses. Anat Rec 155:369–381

Singh RP, Carr DH (1967) Anatomic findings in human abortions of known chromosomal constitution. Obstet Gynecol 29:806

Schenker JG, Weinstein D (1978) Ovarian hyperstimulation syndrome: A current survey. Fertil Steril 30:255–268

Schneider HPG, Hanker JP, Goeser R (1983) Das gestörte Corpus luteum. In: Zander J (ed) Die Sterilität. Urban und Schwarzenberg, München

Starup J, Sele V, Henriksen B (1971) Amenorrhea associated with increased production of gonadotrophins and a morphologically normal ovarian follicular apparatus. Acta Endocrinol 66:248–256

Steiner MM, Hadaw SA (1964) Sexual precocity. Association with follicular cysts of ovary. Am J Dis Child 102:28–36

Sternberg WH, Segaloff A, Gaskill CJ (1953) Influence of chorionic gonadotropin on human ovarian hilus cells (Leydig-like cells). J Clin Endocr 13:139–153

Sternberg WH, Barclay DL (1966) Luteoma of pregnancy. Am J Obstet Gynecol 95:165–185

Stone SL, Pomerantz SH, Schwartz-Kripner A, Channing CP (1978) Biology of Reproduction 19:585–592

Taguchi O, Nishizuka Y, Sakagura T, Kojima A (1980) Autoimmune oophoritis in thymectomized mice: detection of circulating antibodies against oocytes. Clin exp Immunol 40:540–553

Talerman A (1974) Gonadoblastoma associated with embryonal carcinoma. Obstet Gynecol 43:138–142

Talerman A (1980) The pathology of gonadal neoplasms composed of germ cells and sex cord stroma derivations. Path Res Pract 170:24–38

Turner HH (1938) Syndrome of infantilism, congenital webbed neck, and cubitus valgus. Endocrinology 23:566–574

Vandenberg G, Yen SSC (1973) Effect of antiestrogenic action of clomiphene during menstrual cycle: Evidence for change in the feedback sensitivity. J Clin Endocrinol Metab 37:356–365

Vane De GW, Czekala NM, Judd HL, Yen SSC (1975) Circulating gonadotropins, estrogens, and androgens in polycystic ovarian disease. Am J Obstet Gynecol 121:496–500

Vasquez SB, Sotos JF, Kim MH (1982) Massive edema of the ovary and virilization. Obstet Gynecol 59:95S–99S (6 Suppl)

Wachtel SS (1979) The genetics of intersexuality: clinical and theoretic perspectives. Obstet Gynecol 54:671–685

Wentz AC, Jones GS, Sapp KC (1976) Effect of clomiphene citrate on gonadotropin responses to LRH administration in secondary amenorrhea and oligomenorrhea. Obstet Gynecol 47:677–683

Wolf U (1979) Gonadal dysgenesis and the HY-antigen. Report on 12 cases. Hum Genet 47:269–277

Woodcock AS, Govan AD, Gouing NF, Langley FA, Anderson MC (1979) A report of the histological features in 12 cases of gonadoblastoma. Tumori 65:181–189

Woodruff JD, Williams TJ, Goldberg B (1963) Hormone activity of the common ovarian neoplasm. Am J Obstet Gynecol 87:679–698

Young RH, Scully RE (1984) Fibromatosis and massive edema of the ovary, possibly related entities: A report of 14 cases of fibromatosis and 11 cases of massive edema. Int J Gynecol Pathol 3:153–178

Surgical Staging of Ovarian Tumours:
The Individual and Integrative Roles of the Oncologist and Pathologist

L.L. ADCOCK and L.P. DEHNER

Introduction

Ovarian cancer is the leading cause of death in the western world among women with gynecological malignancies. Unfortunately, survival rates for patients with ovarian cancer have not significantly improved in many decades (NORRIS and MURPHY 1932; MOENCH 1933; LYNCH 1936; LINGEMAN 1974; CUTLER et al. 1975). Inasmuch as the majority of patients have advanced clinical stages (FIGO, Stage III or IV) at the time of diagnosis it is not surprising that the overall survival is poor for these unfortunate patients. More discouraging is the fact that at least 30% of the patients with early stage disease, purportedly confined to the ovaries or pelvis, do not survive (BAGLEY et al. 1972). Accurate staging of ovarian cancer, at the initial operative procedure, is essential for planning appropriate treatment for comparing the results of different treatment modalities and for indicating the prognosis (AMERICAN JOINT COMMITTEE 1977; BUCHSBAUM and LIFSHITZ 1984). Understaging unfortunately results in inadequate therapy which in turn compromises an already tentuous clinical situation.

The staging of ovarian cancer is a surgical-pathological procedure and is the only gynecologic malignancy for which the International Federation of Gynecology and Obstetrics (FIGO) requires surgical staging because ovarian malignancies may be confused with gastrointestinal or pancreatic carcinomas. Other gynecological malignancies are staged primarily on the basis of clinical findings without regard for the prognostic features based upon a pathological evaluation. Thus, the surgeon and pathologist both must be knowledgeable about the natural history of ovarian cancer. The surgeon must provide appropriate tissue specimens for histological study of suspected sites of ovarian metastases. A working dialogue is essential in order to diagnose accurately and to stage the disease for optimal patient management and survival. Unfortunately, intraoperative staging for ovarian cancer, particularly in early-stage disease, has too often been incomplete (PIVER et al. 1976; McGOWAN et al. 1985; HELEWA et al. 1986).

1 Dissemination of Ovarian Cancer

Extension of ovarian malignancies to contiguous structures is common and may be microscopic; the ipsilateral fallopian tube, uterus, pelvic peritoneum and adjacent bowel are frequently involved. Malignant cells, once outside of the ovarian neoplasm, circulate throughout the peritoneal cavity (Fig. 1) KEETTEL and ELKINS 1956; MEYERS 1970; MEYERS 1973; KEETTEL et al. 1974; SPINELLI et al. 1976).

Peritoneal fluid has been shown to contain malignant cells when clinical ascites has not been present (KEETTEL and ELKINS 1956). Circulation of the peritoneal fluid in the peritoneal cavity is due to intestinal motility and diaphragmatic respiratory movement. It has long been known that particulate matter in peritoneal fluid implants on the diaphragm (HIGGINS and GRAHAM 1929; OVERHOLT 1931; DYRE 1948; LINDGREN et al. 1968; MEYERS 1970; FELDMAN et al. 1972; FELDMAN and KNAPP 1974). It is somewhat surprising that not until 1973 was attention drawn to the occurrence of diaphragmatic metastases

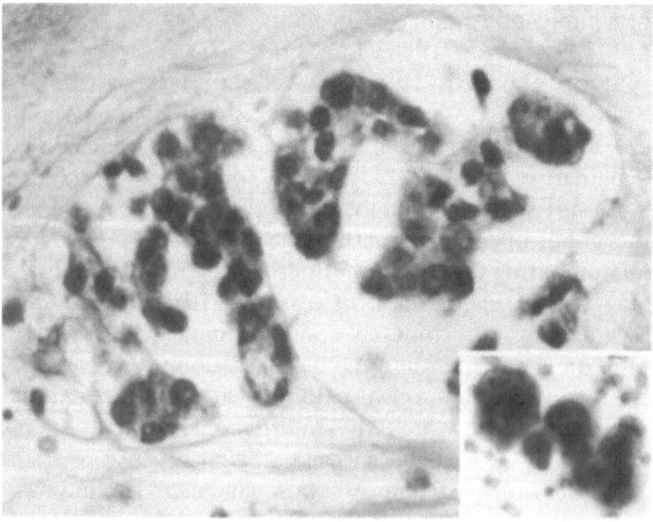

Fig. 1. Clusters and nests of malignant cells from a peritoneal washing obtained at the time of a staging laparotomy in a patient with a presumed stage I-A serous papillary adenocarcinoma. Both the cell block (× 320) and a filter (*inset* × 320) are routinely prepared from the washings

in patients with supposedly early-stage disease. The presence of peritoneal and omental metastases is widely recognized as a common manifestation (MUNNELL 1968; PARKER et al. 1970; KEETTEL et al. 1974; ROSENOFF et al. 1975a; ROSENOFF et al. 1975b; SPINELLI et al. 1976; PIVER et al. 1978).

The significance of lymph node metastases of ovarian cancer has only recently been recognized although the lymphatic drainage of the ovary has been well known (PLENTL and FRIEDMAN 1971; JULIAN et al. 1974; KNAPP and FRIEDMAN 1974; FUKS 1975; CREASMAN et al. 1978; PIVER et al. 1978; MUSUMECI et al. 1980; METZ et al. 1981; CHEN and LEE 1983). Although the main lymphatic pathway from the ovaries has been believed to be the para-aortic lymph nodes, the pelvic lymph nodes are also frequently involved (FUKS 1975; BURGHARDT et al. 1983; CHEN and LEE 1983). Dissemination via the lymph nodes is a frequent route of spread. The histological grade of the neoplasm and the stage of the disease are significant correlates with the incidence of lymph node metastases (WEBB et al. 1973; CHEN and LEE 1983).

2 Primary Surgery

In early stage disease every effort should be made to detect extraovarian and extrapelvic extension, both grossly and microscopically. Thorough histological studies of biopsies of presumed areas of metastases are essential. The more undifferentiated the neoplasm, the more likely that the tumour has or will extend beyond the pelvis (HELEWA et al. 1986). Rupture of the ovarian capsule, when the disease is apparently confined to the ovary, is frequently associated with disease occurring elsewhere during the later clinical course (WEBB et al. 1973; HELEWA et al. 1986). Inasmuch as approximately 30% of the patients who had rupture of the ovarian neoplasm and who had not been adequately staged have more advanced disease, further therapy has been recommended (BAGLEY et al. 1972; FELDMAN and KNAPP 1974; ROSENOFF et al. 1975; SPINELLI et al. 1976; PIVER et al. 1978; YOUNG et al. 1983). Adequate and appropriate staging for patients with true Stage I-A-1 disease can eliminate the necessity for further therapy.

Until recently, the most frequent initial surgical procedure for advanced ovarian cancer was biopsy or limited resection of the neoplasm (TOBIAS and GRIFFITHS 1976; SMITH and DAY 1979; WHARTON and HENSON 1981). The survival rate was dismally low in spite of postoperative chemotherapy and/or radiation therapy. Because of this, evaluation of the results of extensive "cytoreductive" operative procedures, prior to other therapeutic modalities has been in progress with a trend in improved survival rates (GRIFFITHS and FULLER 1978; GRIFFITHS et al. 1979; HANSON et al. 1980; CASTALDO et al. 1981; HACKER et al. 1983; JOYEUX et al. 1986). This improvement of survival following extensive cytoreductive procedures has, however, been questioned (MOORE 1980). It appears that surgically reducing the tumour volume improves the response to chemotherapeutic agents (NELSON 1975; SALMON et al. 1978; GRIFFITHS et al. 1979; SMITH and DAY 1979; HANSON et al. 1980; WHARTON and HENSON 1981;

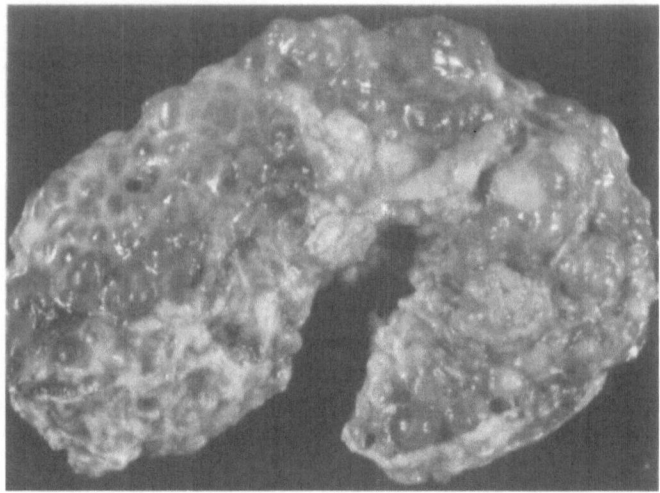

Fig. 2. Omentectomy specimen, showing massive involvement by metastatic serous papillary adeno-carcinoma of the ovary. This procedure was part of cytoreductive therapy. Note the thickened, fibrous and nodular gross appearance of the specimen

JOYEUX et al. 1986). This has been particularly true when cytoreduction was performed at the initial operative procedure (JOYEUX et al. 1986). Extensive cytoreductive surgery for ovarian cancer is a time consuming procedure, with resection of the ovaries, fallopian tubes, uterus, omentum, pelvic peritoneal extension and, not infrequently, bowel resection (CASTALDO et al. 1981; BEREK et al. 1983; COHEN 1985; JOYEUX et al. 1986). Significant morbidity can occur with such procedures (WIJNEN and ROSENSHEIN 1980; BUCHSBAUM and LIFSHITZ 1984). Nonresectable extension of the disease, such as parenchymal liver metastases, retroperitoneal nodal metastases involving small bowel mesentery, involvement of the porta hepatis and/or splenic pedicle, is a contraindication for a radical procedure (WIJNEN 1980; RICHARDSON et al. 1985). Exenteration is rarely indicated for ovarian cancer (BARBER 1983).

The prognosis has been markedly improved when the residual disease is minimal (GRIFFITHS and FULLER 1978; GRIFFITHS et al. 1979; COHEN et al. 1983; COHEN 1985) and is inversely proportional to the amount of residual tumour (DELCLOS and QUINLAN 1969; GRIFFITHS 1975; GRIFFITHS et al. 1979). Such procedures require optimal surgical technique to achieve minimal morbidity. The latter is directly related to the pre-, intra- and postoperative management which frequently involves invasive cardiovascular monitoring and parenteral hyperalimentation (JOYEUX et al. 1986). Ovarian neoplasms apparently confined to the ovary or pelvis require complete staging as a significant percentage have more advanced disease (BAGLEY et al. 1972; KNAPP and FRIEDMAN 1974; PIVER et al. 1978; McGOWAN et al. 1985).

Cytologic evaluation of peritoneal fluid, if present, is mandatory. In the absence of free peritoneal fluid, sterile saline is instilled and later aspirated from the colonic gutters and subdiaphragmatic areas. All peritoneal surfaces, including the diaphragms, are evaluated. Biopsies of all suspicious areas must be obtained. Omentectomy or a large omental biopsy is performed to detect occult metastases (Fig. 2). Should intraoperative frozen section examination fail to identify foci of tumour on the peritoneum or omentum, extensive pelvic, common iliac and para-aortic lymph node sampling is performed. The contralateral ovary, fallopian tube and uterus should be removed in all patients with ovarian cancer with the exception of the young patient in whom the diagnosis is questionable on frozen section (RICHARDSON et al. 1985). This situation is usually a serous or mucinous cystadenoma with a question of borderline malignancy. Reoperation, if indicated, is preferable to unnecessary surgery in such patients (MUNNELL 1969; WILLIAMS and DOCKERTY 1976).

It is mandatory that surgical observations be documented in the operative report and must include an estimate of the volume of ascitic fluid, whether the neoplasm was adherent to other structures, whether the neoplasm had an intact capsule, whether tumour was present on the surface and if ruptured, whether this occurred after obtaining peritoneal cytology. A detailed description of the size and location of tumour masses, both on the initial exploration and at the completion of this procedure, is essential. The surgeon can then review those notes prior to the second-look surgery in order to sample from those approximate same sites during the re-exploration.

3 Second-Look Surgery

This procedure, at the present time, is defined as a surgical exploration when there is no clinical evidence of disease following a prescribed course of therapy (WIJNEN and ROSENSHEIN 1980; COPELAND 1985; CAIN et al. 1986; DAUPLAT et al. 1986; MILLER et al. 1986). The practice of the second-look procedure has evolved as response rates of ovarian malignancies to chemotherapy have improved (SMITH et al. 1972; YOUNG et al. 1978; GRECO et al. 1981; COHEN et al. 1983; RICHARDSON et al. 1985). A clinical impression of a complete response is often negated by the results of the second-look surgery (PHILLIPS et al. 1979; EHRMANN et al. 1980; SCHWARTZ and SMITH 1980; CURRY et al. 1981; GRECO et al. 1981; ROBERTS et al. 1982; STUART et al. 1982; COHEN et al. 1983). Overall, the lower pathological grades and stages of the disease are correlated with a negative second-look operation (RICHARDSON et al. 1985; WALTON et al. 1987). It must be appreciated ever that approximately 10% of all patients with Stage III or Stage IV disease never achieve a negative second-look procedure (SMITH et al. 1976; RAJU et al. 1982; COHEN et al. 1983). A meticulous exploratory laparotomy is the most sensitive method for detection of persistent ovarian carcinoma following therapy. It is the only definitive procedure for identifying those patients who are free of disease or those who have minimal macroscopic or microscopic persistent disease (COHEN 1985; RICHARDSON et al. 1985). Treatment can be discontinued in the former, thereby avoiding further adverse effects, many which are severe, some being fatal (HAYES et al. 1977;

Reiner et al. 1977; Einhorn 1978; Kapadia and Krause 1978; Henderson and Frei 1979).

Unfortunately, noninvasive procedures, such as computerized tomography, ultrasonography, nuclear magnetic resonance imaging, other radiological studies and tumour markers, are insensitive for minimal residual tumour (Amendola et al. 1981; Stern et al. 1981; Mamtora and Isherwood 1982; Goldhirsch et al. 1983; Brenner et al. 1985; Cohen 1985; Nilogg et al. 1985; Clarke-Pearson et al. 1986). Laparoscopy is of value if persistent disease can be confirmed by biopsy (Mangioni et al. 1979; Berek et al. 1981). Laparotomy is necessary in all other situations. Peritoneal fluid, if present, is submitted for cytological examination; otherwise sterile saline is instilled and later aspirated from peritoneal gutters and subdiaphragmatic areas. Extensive histological sampling, ranging from 30 to 50 biopsies, of the sites of previous disease, peritoneum of the cul-de-sac, pelvis and colonic gutters and hemidiaphragms, is necessary. Should cancer not be identified, resection of the remaining infundibulopelvic ligaments, omentectomy or resection of the remaining omentum and extensive sampling of the pelvic and para-aortic lymph nodes are indicated. It cannot be too strongly emphasized that occult metastases can be present without visual or palpable abnormalities. Scrapings of the hemidiaphragms for cytology are of value.

Second-look surgery, without gross evidence of disease, is a time-consuming, meticulous procedure; it is therefore contraindicated in certain situations, such as severe medical complications and extensive intraabdominal adhesions, because of the high risk of complications. Second-look surgery, overall, has low morbidity and minimal mortality (Roberts et al. 1982; Webb et al. 1982; Cain et al. 1986).

Unfortunately, there is no guarantee against recurrence following a negative second-look exploration when residual, persistent or recurrent tumour has not been identified (Copeland and Gershenson 1986). The lower the initial stage prior to the negative second-look procedure, the less likely is recurrent disease (Phillips et al. 1979; Cain et al. 1986). When Stage III or IV disease was initially present, the recurrence rate following negative second-look surgery ranges from 14 to 33% (Curry et al. 1981; Stuart et al. 1982; Webb et al. 1982; Budd et al. 1983; Gershenson et al. 1985; Cain et al. 1986; Young 1987).

4 Reoperation for Ovarian Cancer

Reoperation, prior to chemotherapy or radiation therapy, may be indicated when a suboptimal initial operation was performed. Surgery is frequently necessary in the presence of progressive disease for relief of bowel obstruction. The value of more extensive resection of tumour, after partial response to chemotherapy, is somewhat controversial, although in selected patients it has been beneficial (Berek et al. 1982; Cain et al. 1986).

5 Pathological Examination

The extraordinary thoroughness of the surgical procedure requires an equally fastidious pathological examination of the specimens. Of course, the containers received in the surgical pathology laboratory should be carefully labeled in the surgical suite. Lapses occur on occasion and the consequence is uncertainty about the sites of the multitudinous biopsies. It is counterproductive for the surgeon to spend the time and effort in a careful exploration only to have the information compromised through a clerical error. In a patient with peritoneal carcinomatosis, there is less concern about the specific location but in the presence of very limited microscopic disease, the clinician is considerably more interested since it may point to areas where additional therapy may be directed (DI SAIA and CREASMAN 1984).

These specimens are often small, measuring only a few millimeters, and for that reason they should be submitted *en toto* and even stained with hematoxylin by the prosector so that the histotechnologist is better able to visualize the tissue during the processing procedure. Multiple levels from the block are suggested in order to avoid the possibility of overlooking a focus of neoplastic tissue. Lymph nodes may harbor a few malignant glands in the subcapsular sinuses so that several levels are recommended in order to facilitate their detection. Our own experience is that 5% of nodal metastases would have gone undetected if deeper levels had not been obtained and carefully examined. Once all of the tissue has been reviewed microscopically, an attempt should be made to semiquantitate the amount of tumour based upon the number of positive peritoneal biopsies and lymph nodes. Also, a comment should be made about the tumour in terms of the degree of involvement in each biopsy so as to convey some impression about the "tumour load" with the realization that this assesment is a very broad approximation but nonetheless a helpful one in some cases.

5.1 Histological Features of the Metastases at Initial Surgery

Of course, the histological type and grade of the ovarian malignancy are central parameters to the prognosis (JULIAN et al. 1974; MALKASIAN et al. 1975; HART 1981; RUSSELL 1987). The classification which we apply is the one proposed by the World Health Organization and discussed by LANGLEY and FOX (1987). An entry in this classification which has not received very much attention in the literature is the "mixed epithelial tumour"; our experience is that 10% or so of malignant "common epithelial tumours" have more than one distinctive epithelial pattern.

Metastases to the peritoneum and omentum or within lymph nodes at the initial surgical resection invariably recapitulate the pathological grade and tumour type of the primary ovarian neoplasm (Fig. 3) (CHEN and LEE 1983). The exceptions in some cases include the mixed mullerian tumour whose metastatic lesions may consist predominantly or exclusively of the carcinomatous

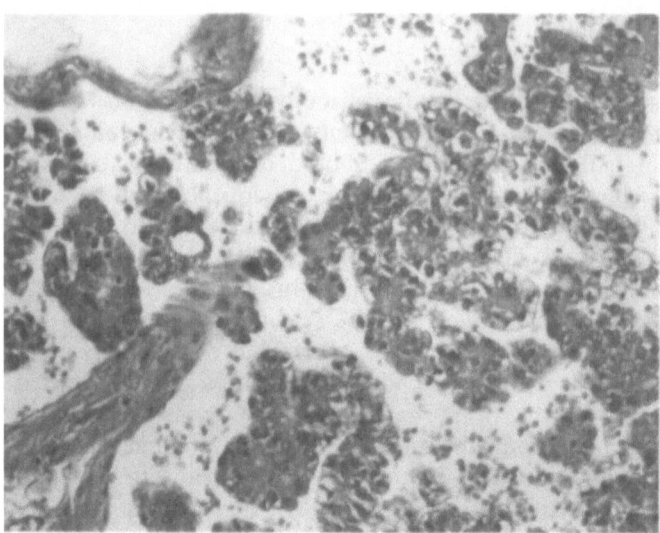

Fig. 3. Peritoneal metastasis of a clear cell or mesonephroid carcinoma, showing a papillary pattern and the characteristic clear cell cytology, × 128

or sarcomatous component (Fig. 4) or a mixed malignant germ cell tumour with only teratomatous elements in the metastases. In the latter case, it is difficult to predict the nature of the metastasis and its histological grade; a mature or partially immature teratoma can have differentiated glial implants or gliomatosis peritonei or immature neuroepithelium (Heydenrych et al. 1979; Nielsen et al. 1985). Norris et al. (1976) have emphasized the importance of grading the peritoneal metastases histologically. Nodal gliomatosis is another seemingly innocuous form of involvement by a solid teratoma (Perrone et al. 1986). However, the rare mature cystic teratoma may undergo malignant transformation with squamous cell carcinoma in the pelvis or elsewhere in the peritoneal cavity. There is a small subset of surface papillary tumours with diffuse intraabdominal neoplasia and small ovaries. Microscopic foci of tumour are present on the surface of the ovaries and implants are found on the parietes (Fig. 5). Multifocal primary tumours have been suggested in lieu of metastases from the ovaries (August et al. 1985; Russell et al. 1985).

5.2 Intraoperative Frozen Section Examination

The intraoperative frozen section examination is an important adjunct to the surgeon on occasion so that a pathological diagnosis can be established if possible at the time of the procedure (Silva 1987). If there is no macroscopic evidence of spread beyond the ovary from a suspected malignancy, it is obviously important to determine whether the unilateral or bilateral ovarian mass(es) is indeed neoplastic. A functional cyst (follicular or theca-lutein cyst), mature cystic teratoma or an endometriotic cyst will be approached in a conservative manner,

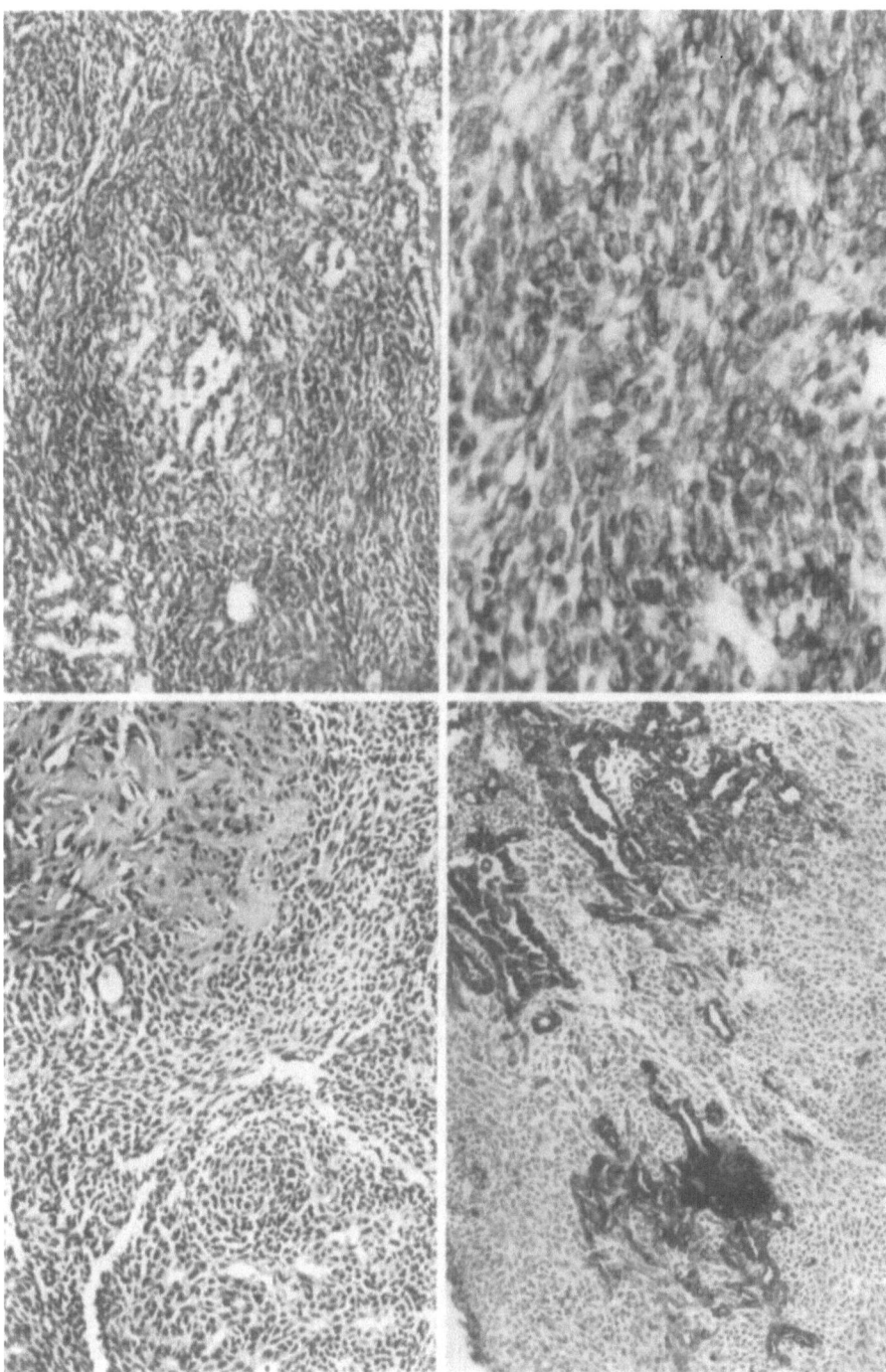

Fig. 4. Mixed mullerian tumour of the ovary, showing the predominantly spindle cell sarcomatous appearance with only focal poorly formed glands in the primary tumour (*upper left*, ×128) and vimentin immunoreactivity of the spindle cells (*upper right*, ×315). Although the peritoneal metastases also had a sarcomatous quality (*lower left*, ×128), the cytokeratin immunoreactivity demonstrated the adenocarcinomatous component (*lower right*, ×128)

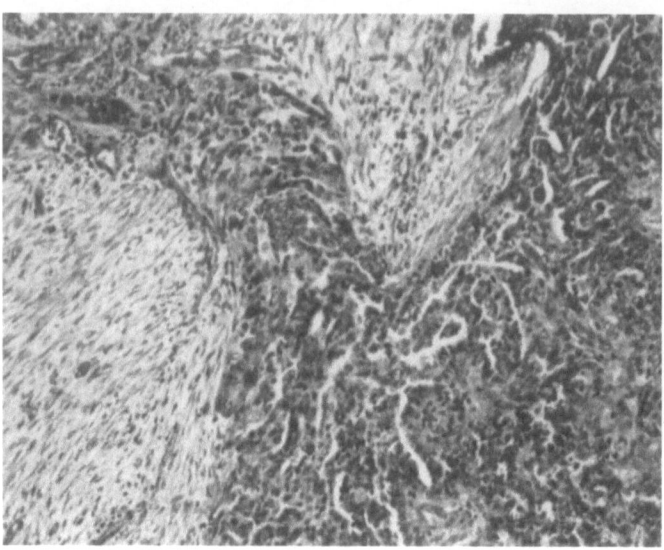

Fig. 5. Serous papillary adenocarcinoma, showing extensive peritoneal seeding yet there was only superficial microscopic involvement of the ovaries, × 128

whereas an overt malignancy will receive the appropriate surgical attention which was described in the preceding sections of this discussion.

When there is a suspicion that the mass is malignant from gross inspection at surgery, an oophorectomy is usually performed and submitted for pathological evaluation. A careful examination of the external surface may identify irregularities or excrescences possibly indicating that the capsule has been penetrated by tumour. In the absence of any capsular abnormalities, the mass should be measured, weighed and opened carefully so that the liquid contents can be collected for a volumetric determination and qualitative characterization. We have not routinely filtered the fluid for cytology since much of it is inadvertently lost no matter how delicately the specimen is entered. Once the specimen has been bisected, papillary and solid areas if present should be sampled (Fig. 6). Touch imprints of suspicious areas are obtained, immediately fixed in 70% ethanol and stained in haematoxylin and eosin concurrently with the frozen sections. The cytological detail is often far superior in the touch imprints than in the usual frozen sections. There are practical limitations in the extent of the intraoperative pathological examination in terms of the tissue sampling especially in the presence of a large mass. Localized areas of capsular invasion may not be appreciated; this is a particular problem in the low grade surface papillary neoplasms (borderline malignant serous or mucinous cystadenoma). A prototypic clinical situation is the young woman between 20 and 35 years of age with bilateral masses of a borderline type and there is the desire to preserve some ovarian function or even fertility. These are the moments that test the collegeality between the surgeon and pathologist and ultimately the trust of the surgeon in the pathologist.

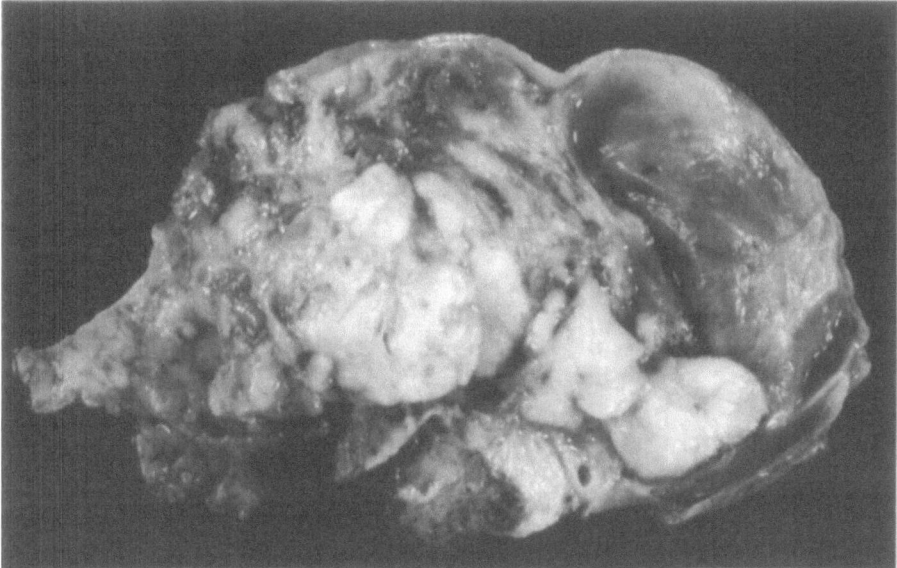

Fig. 6. An ovarian mass with this appearance on cross section generally evokes few problems in the determination of malignancy. Because of the solid and cystic nature of this tumour, an endometroid carcinoma was a consideration, however, the histology revealed a malignant Brenner tumour

Once the pathological diagnosis of an ovarian malignancy has been settled, the question of a primary or a metastatic neoplasm may arise, particularly in the contexts of a mucinous adenocarcinoma, signet ring cell carcinoma or a carcinoid tumour (ROBBOY et al. 1974; ROBBOY et al. 1975; LASH and HART 1987). There are some histological distinctions between the primary carcinoid of the ovary which is generally regarded as a monodermal teratoma and the metastatic carcinoid usually from a primary site in the small intestine. Those nuances may or may not be apparent intraoperatively to the surgeon or pathologist. A careful inspection of the terminal ileum and sampling of mesenteric lymph nodes may provide the clues for the resolution of the dilemma. Signet ring carcinoma of the ovary typically occurs bilaterally and fulfills the criterion for Krukenberg tumours (HOLTZ and HART 1982; ULBRIGHT and ROTH 1985). However, the stromal component of the background may obscure the presence of the signet ring cells resulting in the diagnosis of a sex cord-mesenchyme neoplasm such as a fibroma-thecoma with luteinized cells. A touch imprint of the freshly sectioned surface may circumvent this potential error with the succesful identification of signet ring cells. However, the surgeon should be suspicious of the diagnosis of bilateral sex cord-mesenchyme neoplasms and gently challenge the pathologist's interpretation. Another category of non-ovarian malignancies involving the ovaries is the haematolymphoid proliferations including acute leukaemia and non-Hodgkin's lymphoma (YOUNG and SCULLY 1987). Small non-cleaved cell (Burkitt's and non-Burkitt's types) and large cleaved cell lymphomas are the major subtypes affecting the ovaries (Fig. 7)

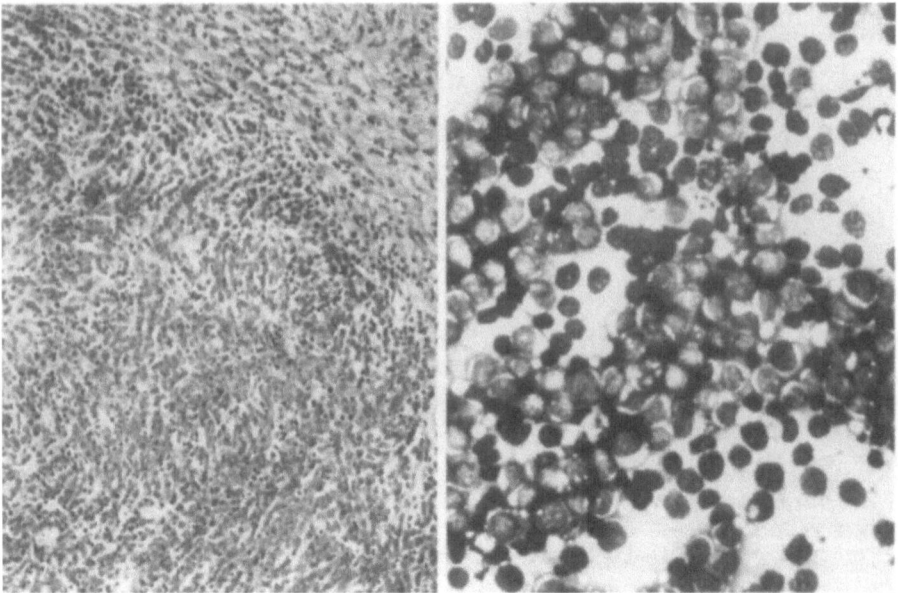

Fig. 7. Malignant lymphoma, small non-cleaved cell (non-Burkitt's type), presenting as pelvic masses in a 22-year-old woman. At surgery, both ovaries were enlarged and a biopsy of one showed cord-like profiles of small hyperchromatic cells (*left*, × 110) which suggested the possibility of small cell carcinoma or stromal neoplasm. A touch imprint (*right*, × 276) unequivocally demonstrated the lymphoid nature of the tumour cells which later were shown to be B-lymphocytes

(CHORLTON 1987). There are rare examples of primary lymphoma of the ovary (PIURA et al. 1986), but most cases are a manifestation of widespread abdominal disease with retroperitoneal lymphadenopathy if not more generalized involvement. When a mucinous cystadenoma or adenocarcinoma of the ovary presents on the right side, careful palpation of the appendix, cecum and ascending colon is indicated (MERINO et al. 1985). Histopathologically, the mucinous adenocarcinoma of the ovary and colon has many features in common. In the case of synchronous or metachronous mucinous adenocarcinoma of the ovary and colon, the determination of the primary sites should rely upon such factors as the pathological stage of the colonic neoplasm, in particular the status of the mesenteric lymph nodes. It is better in our estimation to sort through these issues after a thorough pathological examination rather than during surgery, but occasionally some matters require an intraoperative solution or an attempt at one. As a final note on the subject of metastasis to the ovaries, neuroblastoma, rhabdomyosarcoma and malignant melanoma are infrequently encountered.

Surgical staging of ovarian cancer begins at the point when the pathologist transmits the frozen section diagnosis to the surgeon or the surgeon initiates the process when it is obvious from an inspection of the pelvis (BUCHSBAUM and LIFSHITZ 1984; DISAIA and CREASMAN 1984; GRIFFITHS and PARKER 1986). Biopsies of the peritoneum are submitted to establish the presence of suspected

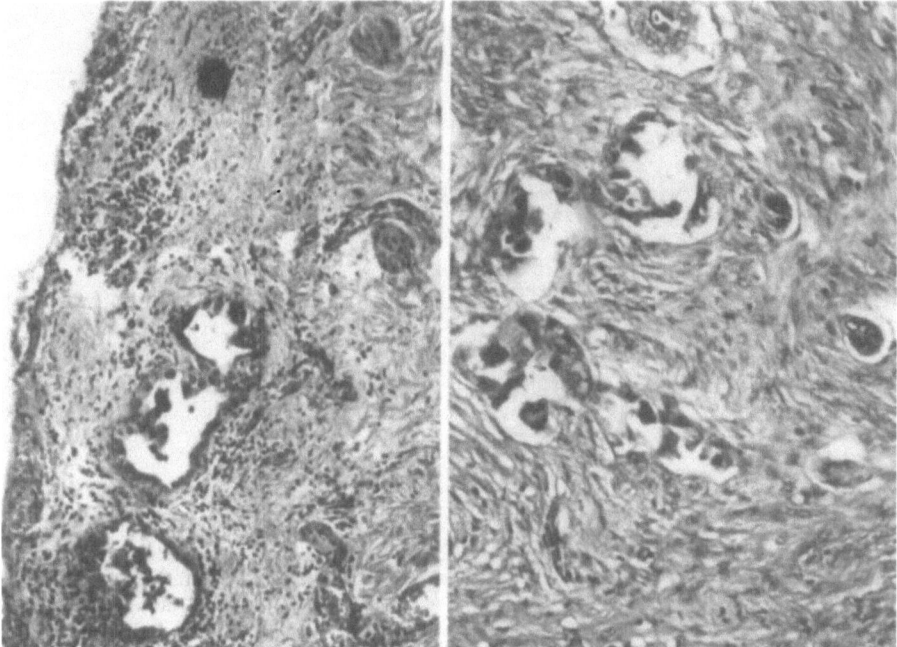

Fig. 8. Two representative peritoneal biopsies, showing glandular proliferations immediately beneath the surface mesothelium (*left*, × 126) with minimal reaction in the stroma and an isolated psammoma body. The marked cytologic atypia of the glands was regarded as sufficient for a diagnosis of metastatic adenocarcinoma. Psammoma bodies *per se* in the biopsy are not diagnostic of malignancy. Another biopsy (*right*, × 126) with neoplastic glands had the characteristic desmoplastic stroma

malignant implants or to determine the status of the parietes in the questionable case (Fig. 8). The interpretation of these specimens is usually straightforward with the exception of the fatty biopsy which is negative for tumour in the majority of cases or of the biopsy with proliferative changes on the surface which may represent reactive mesothelial hyperplasia or endosalpingiosis, however, uncertainty may exist at frozen section and only the permanent sections have the potential for resolving the point (FARHI and SILVERBERG 1982; MC CAUGHEY 1985; MICHAEL and ROTH 1986). Intraoperative lymph node examination is tedious and has the risk of transmitting a "false negative" impression. For instance, metastatic tumour may appear on permanent section in deeper levels of the lymph node(s) which was not present in the original frozen section and appropriately interpreted as "negative for malignancy". Smaller lymph nodes in the mesentery or retroperitoneal soft tissues may be overlooked during the intraoperative pathologic evaluation and only become apparent after fixation and clearing of the entire specimen (CHEN and LEE 1983; WU et al. 1986). Benign glandular inclusions in a lymph node is a potential source of error for a "false positive" interpretation of metastatic adenocarcinoma (Fig. 9) (EHRMANN et al. 1980; HSU et al. 1980; FARHI and SILVERBERG 1982).

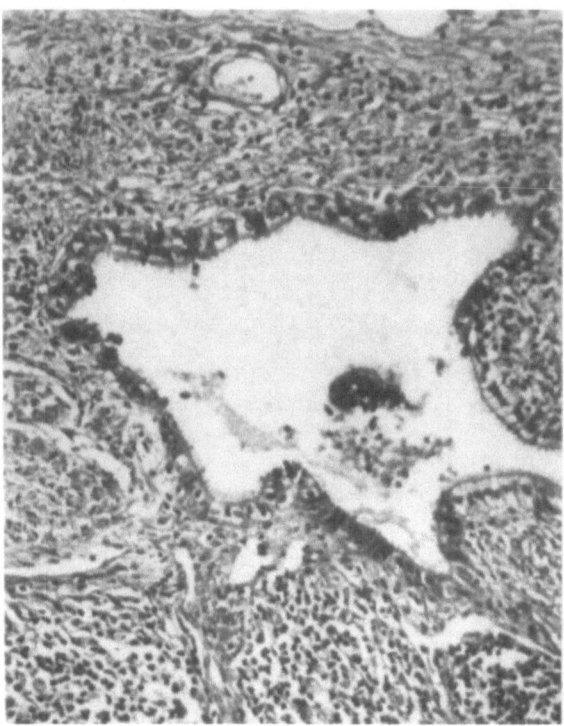

Fig. 9. Benign glandular inclusion or endosalpingiosis of the lymph node, showing a single gland in the capsule. The single layer of columnar epithelial cells has a ciliated surface, ×142

5.3 Post-Surgical Pathological Examination

A period of fixation is preferred in our laboratory before the specimen is examined since blocks can be obtained with greater ease but it creates a delay in the final report by a day or so. Tissue is obtained immediately for electron microscopy and flow cytometry, and the fresh specimen is photographed. One rapidly processed gross illustration is used by the prosector to label the location of the blocks for microscopic examination. There is no set formula for the number of sections per centimeter or weight of tumour, but generally 10 or more sections from the ovarian mass are taken. Extensive sampling of the capsule to identify foci of invasion and surface involvement is necessary because of its impact upon the final clinicopathological staging of the tumour (OZOLS and YOUNG 1987). Multiple histological sections also provide the opportunity to study any variations in the histological pattern(s) and pathological grade. For instance, the majority of surface epithelial derived malignancies are serous papillary adenocarcinomas; the higher pathological grades (grade III–IV) are often solid with only focal papillary areas if present at all. Other benefits of a thorough pathological examination of an ovarian malignancy is the identification of homologous or heterologous sarcomatous elements (mixed mullerian tumour), mixed patterns of carcinoma (endometrioid, clear cell or mesonephroid and mucinous foci) and minor areas of anaplasia. Some of the solid tumours may present the differential diagnostic problem of an adenocarcinoma of surface origin or a granulosa cell tumour. Small gland-like spaces within the solid nests may suggest the formation of Call-Exner bodies. More often than not, these large solid neoplasms are poorly differentiated adenocarcinomas, but immuno-histochemistry is potentially helpful since the granulosa cell tumour typically expresses vimentin in the cytoplasm and the carcinomas are reactive for cytoker-atin, epithelial membrane antigen, amylase and CA-125 (NOUWEN et al. 1987). A simple resolution is to examine the cells for nuclear grooves in the suspected granulosa cell tumour; parenthetically, the fold in the nuclear membrane is also present in the proliferating and malignant Brenner tumours.

The differential diagnosis of a mucinous adenocarcinoma in the ovary was addressed in an earlier section but a more common problem is the large contiguous adnexal-uterine neoplasm in which case, the issue is one of the ovarian versus fundic origin of the tumour; the fallopian tube is another yet less frequent possibility. It should be appreciated at the onset that the issue is not settled in every case to everybody's satisfaction since it is a matter of interpretation of a set of findings which is subject to alternative scenarios. One important factor for differing conclusions is the overlapping histological patterns of uterine and ovarian carcinomas of virtually all types including the "endometrioid" adenocarcinoma, mixed mullerian tumour and serous papillary adenocarcinoma. Secondly, the bulky replacement of both organs renders an accurate assessment of the exact primary site very difficult. If peritoneal spread is prominent or if the contralateral ovary is involved by a similar appearing surface-derived epithelial tumour, then the ovary is the logical primary site. When the uterus contains an unequivocal adenocarcinoma with an endometrial component and one that has convincingly arisen from the surface, the conclusion is that the "endometrioid" carcinoma in the ovary originated in the uterus; this principle regarding endometrioid carcinoma has prevailed for many years (CZERNOBILSKY 1985). In fact, primary endometrioid carcinoma of the ovary was accepted without qualifications in those cases without a primary endometrial carcinoma or if one was present, it was confined to the endometrium (Fig. 10). Hormone receptor studies and immunohistochemistry are not entirely reliable nor sufficiently specific to differentiate between ovarian and endometrial carcinoma. A thoughtful discussion between the clinician and pathologist about the findings is the more likely method to resolve any residual questions.

The pathological distinction of the so-called borderline malignant serous or mucinous cystadenoma from the well-differentiated serous or mucinous cyst-adenocarcinoma is a source of continuing consternation as judged from our own experience and the literature (COLGAN and NORRIS 1983; HOPKINS et al. 1987). Approximately 25%–30% of the borderline serous tumours are bilateral and less than 10% of the mucinous counterparts involve both ovaries (Fig. 11). Peritoneal extension is a not uncommon feature of the borderline serous cyst-adenomas; papillary and/or glandular structures are present on the surface of the ovary and peritoneum. Whether the surface neoplasm is an adenocarcinoma or a borderline malignancy, the metastatic deposits should be qualified as invading the peritoneum or serosa or localized within a superficial fibrous or desmoplastic reaction (Fig. 12) (MICHAEL and ROTH 1986). The borderline mucinous

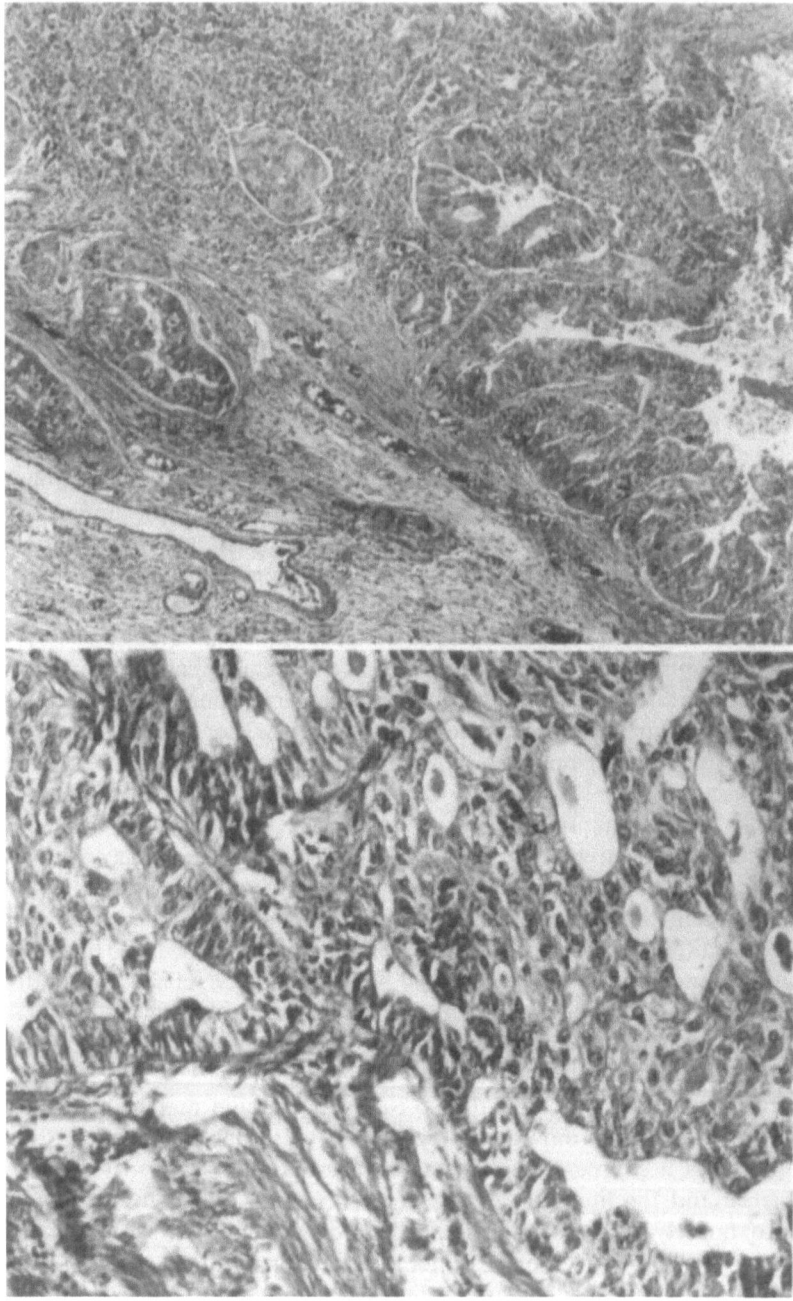

Fig. 10. Moderately differentiated adenocarcinoma (FIGO, grade II) with endometrioid pattern replacing the adnexal region (*top*, × 64) and invading into the myometrium (*bottom*, × 400. Exentive sampling failed to establish a primary site in the endometrium. The ovary in this case was the origin of an endometrioid carcinoma

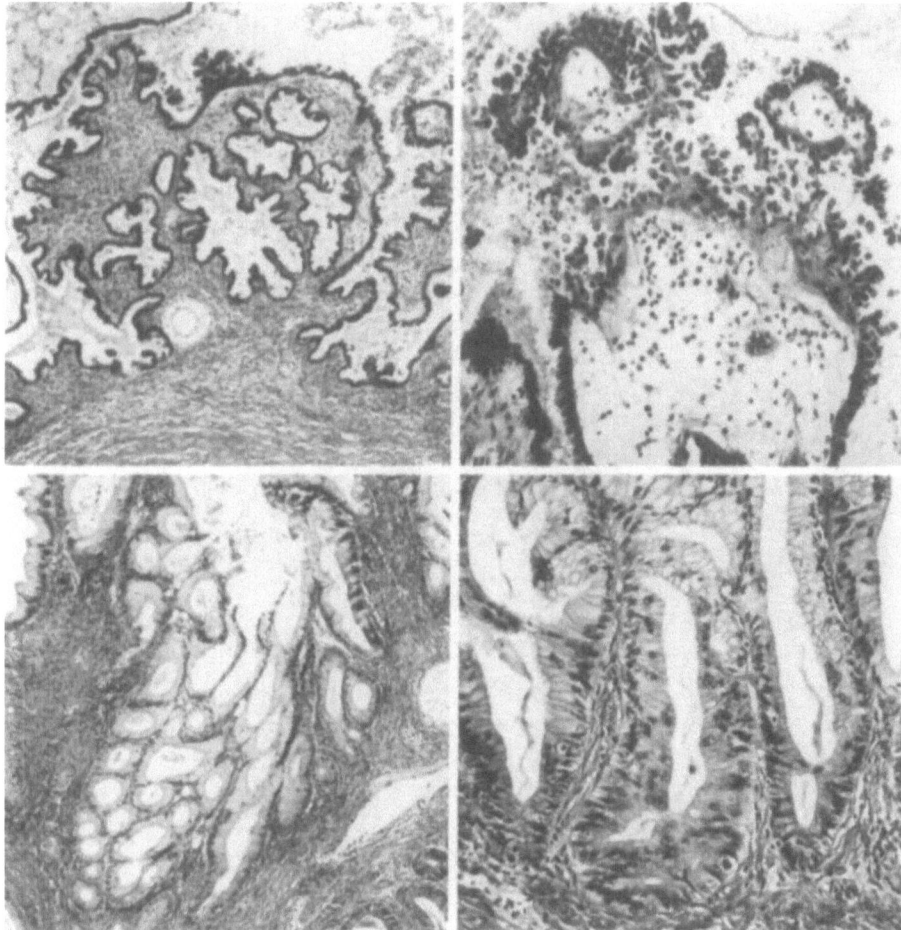

Fig. 11. Composite illustration of a borderline malignant serous (*top, left and right,* ×45) and mucinous (*bottom, left* and *right,* ×115) cystadenoma. One of the major problems in pathologic differential diagnosis concerns the presence or absence of stromal invasion which is the discriminating feature between the borderline and overtly malignant surface papillary epithelial neoplasm

cystadenoma may be accompanied by a mucinous cystadenoma of the appendix. Localized extra-ovarian acellular mucinous extravasation does not connote malignancy but if neoplastic cells are found within pools of mucin, this is regarded as evidence of a mucinous adenocarcinoma. The gross appearance of a borderline malignant cystadenoma does not vary substantially from its carcinomatous counterpart which is not surprising given the fact that the microscopic differences are marginal. Unlike the unilocular serous cystadenoma with a smooth or velvety surface or the multiloculated mucinous cystadenoma with its equally innocuous appearance, the borderline variants have focal or diffuse papillae on the internal surface of the cyst. Firm nodules in the wall of the cyst or projecting into the cyst are present in those tumours with a "fibromatous"

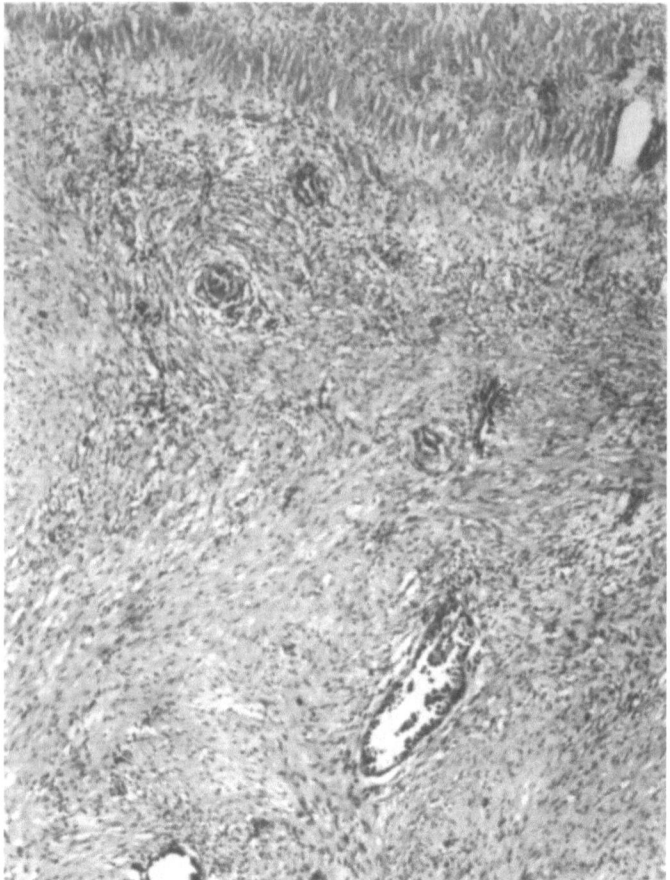

Fig. 12. Borderline malignant serous cystadenoma, showing metastatic deposits in a thickened desmoplastic stroma on the serosal surface of the small intestine. There was no evidence of direct invasion into the bowel wall, × 64

component in which case the neoplasm is a cystadenofibroma (Fig. 13). Microscopically, the papillae of the borderline tumour have a complex, often branching and tufting configuration and are supported by variable amounts of fibrovascular stroma (Fig. 11). Those papillae with a prominent stroma are often associated with fibrous thickening of the capsule; these features are indicative of a cystadenofibroma. Cellular stratification, cytological atypia without anaplasia and occasional mitoses are the principal epithelial abnormalities (Fig. 11). Giant cells and bizarre mitoses are typically absent. The complicated papillary structures may produce deep clefts into the wall of the cyst with an appearance simulating capsular invasion; it is basically the presence or absence of invasion exclusive of other features which differentiates the borderline malignant tumour from a low-grade cystadenocarcinoma. This still does not explain the source of the peritoneal implants in the case of the non-invasive borderline malignant

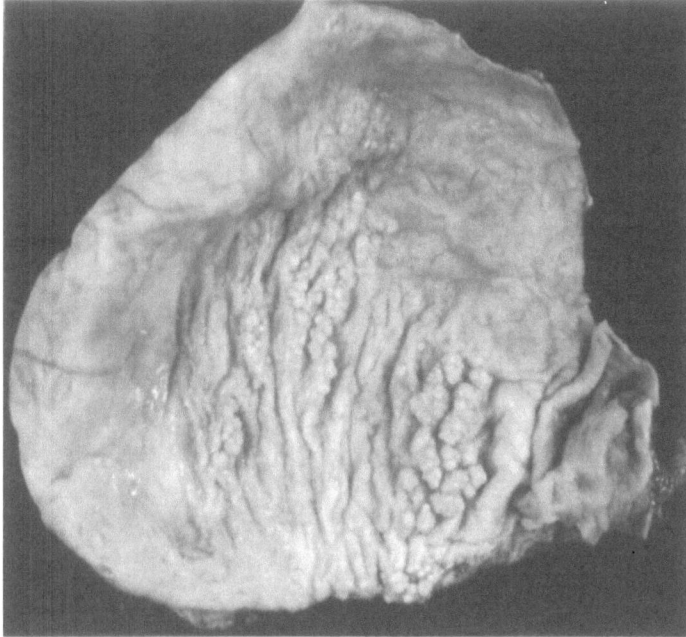

Fig. 13. Borderline malignant serous cystadenoma, showing papillary irregularities on the cyst wall after the large unilocular cyst has been opened. Many of the papillary excrescences had a prominent fibrous stroma

tumour. Parenthetically, the peritoneal implants of a borderline mucinous tumour are more often than not localized to the region of the involved ovary whereas the peritoneum is diffusely studded by the borderline serous tumour. Only 2%–5% of patients with a borderline malignant tumour succumb to tumour, but it is a measure that these neoplasms are malignant both clinically and pathologically (BOSTWICK et al. 1986).

6 Pathology of the Second-Look Operation

Many of the problems which the pathologist is likely to encounter in the examination of biopsies from the second-look operation are to be found among the first-look cases. For instance, the metastases may have a different histological appearance from the primary tumour producing some concern about the possibility of a second primary neoplasm. In most cases, the metastatic lesions closely resemble the original tumour even in those situations of a sex cord-mesenchyme tumour like the granulosa cell tumour (Fig. 14). The added difficulties are a consequence of the initial intra-abdominal surgical procedure, response of tumour to therapy and possible reaction of normal tissues to chemotherapy and/or irradiation.

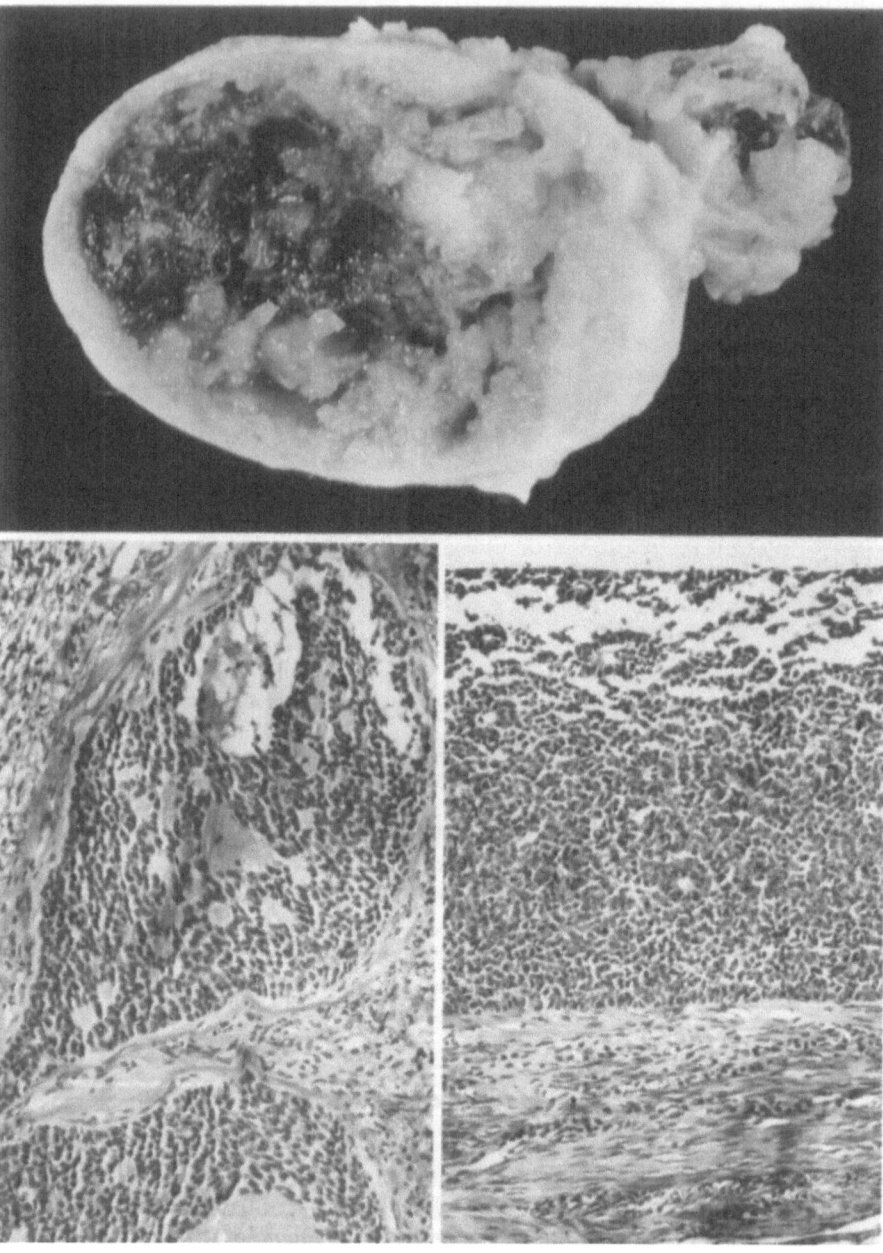

Fig. 14. Granulosa cell tumour, showing a cystic and partially hemorrhagic metastasis (*top*) discovered at the time of a second-look laparotomy. A representative microscopic field of the primary tumour (*bottom left*, ×130) is compared with the metastasis (*bottom right*, ×130). Call-Exner bodies were easily found in the primary tumour, but only small rosette-like profiles were evident in the metastasis

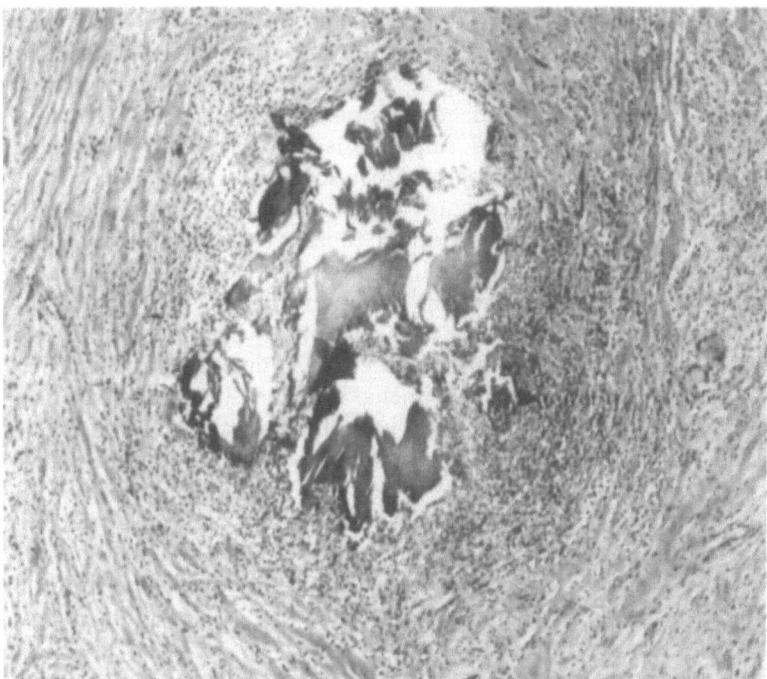

Fig. 15. Foreign body with a granulomatous reaction in several peritoneal biopsies obtained at a second-look laparotomy. The clinical impression at surgery was recurrent carcinoma, × 64

Our experience with the cyto- and histopathological findings in the second-look operation was reported in a study of 85 cases (COFFIN et al. 1985). These patients had achieved a clinical remission at 9–12 months and had completed the chemotherapy before the second-look procedure. Very few of the patients had manifestations of a suspected recurrence at the time of surgery. Four basic diagnostic categories were applied to the histological and cytological findings: negative for malignancy, negative with benign atypia, negative with benign glandular inclusions and endosalpingiosis and unequivocally positive for malignancy. Approximately 25% of the patients had biopsy-proven recurrent or persistent malignancy and 40% of the cases were entirely negative for malignancy. The remaining biopsies showed "benign atypia" which included mesothelial hyperplasia, psammoma bodies without accompanying epithelium, focal peritoneal necrosis with a foreign body giant cell reaction and focal fibroblastic-myofibroblastic proliferation simulating a fibrous histiocytoma or fibrous mesothelioma (Fig. 15). All of these lesions were microscopic findings.

Atypical mesothelial hyperplasia, endosalpingiosis and benign glandular inclusions were the problematic findings occurring in approximately 5% of cases. Mesothelial hyperplasia is recognized by the presence of a prominent single layer of mesothelial cells with focal tufts of cells on the surface. In contrast, atypical hyperplasia is a markedly proliferative process with stratification of mesothelial cells and papillary projections. Mesothelial cells may be found in the immediate zone of fibrosis beneath the surface as individual polygonal and spindle-shaped cells. However, deep invasion into the subperitoneal connective tissues or fat of the omentum should be regarded as evidence of malignancy and in the case of a known papillary adenocarcinoma, the diagnostic conclusion is straightforward in most cases. Endosalpingiosis and the benign glandular inclusions are very likely related histogenetically in some cases since both lesions are present in the same patient. In a study by ZINSSER and WHEELER (1982), chronic inflammatory disease of the fallopian tubes was found in each case so that the possibility of benign epithelial implants was a consideration. These authors dismissed the metaplasia hypothesis or endometriosis which we personally favor. The glands are often solitary and surrounded by a fibrous stroma but without the condensed cellular appearance of endometrial stroma as in endometriosis. One or several layers of epithelial cells may line the glands and some degree of nuclear hyperchromasia is not infrequent. Ideally, the cell surface should be ciliated. Papillary infoldings and psammoma bodies are other findings. A desmoplastic reaction around the glands should be viewed with concern about the possibility of metastatic adenocarcinoma. An especially difficult problem is the one of a borderline malignant serous cystadenoma with extensive glandular and papillary profiles in the omental and peritoneal specimen. The biopsies may disclose a spectrum of findings from endosalpingiosis to borderline malignant implants.

Benign glandular inclusions in the lymph nodes are typically found in the capsule rather than in the subcapsular sinusoids or isolated within the node without a discernible relationship to the sinuses. The glands are usually solitary or occasionally multiple and have a more or less uniform, round to oval contour. An open lumen with or without secretions, small papillations, and luminal psammoma bodies are additional features. The epithelial cells have bland cytologic features including a low nuclear-cytoplasmic ratio, delicate chromatin pattern, and absence of mitoses. When cytologic atypia is present in suspected glandular inclusions, this is attributed to the effects of the cytotoxic chemotherapy. In the doubtful case, we have found that a selected panel of immunohistochemical stains are useful. Although cytokeratin, epithelial membrane antibody and human milk fat globule protein were expressed in benign glandular inclusions and metastatic carcinoma, carcinoembryonic antigen (CEA) and Leu M1 were respectively specific and sensitive for malignancy (MANIVEL et al. 1988). DIENEMANN and PICKARTZ (1987) in a similar immunohistochemical study on peritoneal implants of ovarian carcinoma did not find that CEA was a useful marker. We are unable to immediately explain the discrepancy in our respective results and conclusions.

7 Epilogue

Thorough clinicopathological staging of ovarian tumours is essential to accurate prognostic assessment and the formulation of a treatment plan. With the exception of some types of malignant lymphoma, there is probably no other group of malignancies which is subjected to such a rigorous and formalized scheme of surgical staging followed by histopathological verification as an ovary cancer. This discussion has attempted to convey the necessity for a close working dialogue between the oncologist and pathologist from the time that the surgeon takes the first specimen. There are many opportunities and circumstances for problems to arise and the resolution often relies upon the ability of the clinician and pathologist to communicate in order to best serve the needs of the patient. The authors are well aware of the pitfalls and have shared some of our insights in this review.

References

Amendola MA, Walsh JW, Amendola BE, Tisnado J, Hall DJ, Goplerud DR (1981) Computed tomography in the evaluation of carcinoma of the ovary. J Comput Assist Tomogr 5:179–186

American Joint Committee for Cancer Staging and End-Results Reporting (1977) Manual for Staging of Cancer. Chicago

August CZ, Murad TM, Newton M (1985) Multiple focal extraovarian serous carcinoma. Int J Gynecol Pathol 4:11–23

Bagley CM Jr, Young RC, Canellos GP, DeVita VT (1972) The treatment of ovarian carcinoma: possibilities for progress. N Engl J Med 287:856–862

Bagley CM, Young RC, Schein PS, Chabner BA, DeVita VT (1973) Ovarian carcinoma metastatic to the diaphragms – frequently undiagnosed at laparotomy. Am J Obstet Gynecol 116:397–400

Barber HRK (1983) The role of surgery in carcinoma of the ovary. Bull NY Acad Med 59:276–287

Berek JS, Griffiths CT, Leventhal JM (1981) Laparoscopy for second-look evaluation in ovarian cancer. Gynecol Oncol 7:47–55

Berek JS, Hacker NF, Lagasse LD, Leuchter RS (1982) Lower urinary tract resection as part of cytoreductive surgery for ovarian cancer. Gynecol Oncol 13:87–92

Berek JS, Hacker NF, Lagasse LD, Nieberg RK, Elashoff RM (1983) Survival of patients following secondary cytoreductive surgery in ovarian cancer. Obstet Gynecol 61:189–193

Bostwick DG, Tazelaar HD, Ballon SC, Hendrickson MR, Kempson RL (1986) Ovarian epithelial tumors of borderline malignancy. A clinical and pathologic study of 109 cases. Cancer 58:2052–2065

Brenner DE, Shaff MI, Jones HW, Grosh WW, Greco FA, Burnett LS (1985) Abdominopelvic computed tomography: evaluation in patients undergoing second-look laparotomy for ovarian carcinoma. Obstet Gynecol 65:715–717

Buchsbaum HJ, Lifshitz S (1984) Staging and surgical evaluation of ovarian cancer. Semin Oncol 11:227–237

Budd GT, Webster KD, Reimer RR, Martimbeau P, Livingston RB (1983) Treatment of advanced ovarian cancer with cisplatin, adriamycin, and cyclophosphamide. Effect of treatment and incidence of intracranial metastases. J Surg Oncol 24:192–195

Burghardt E, Pickel H, Holzer E, Lahousen M (1983) The significance of lymphadenectomy in therapy of ovarian carcinoma. Am J Obstet Gynecol 146:111–112

Cain JM, Saigo PE, Pierce VK, Clark DG, Jones WB, Smith DH, Hakes TB, Ochoa M, Lewis JL (1986) A review of second-look laparotomy for ovarian cancer. Gynecol Oncol 23:14–25

Castaldo TW, Petrilli ES, Ballon SC, Lagasse LD (1981) Intestinal operations in patients with ovarian cancer. Am J Obstet Gynecol 139:80–84

Chen SS, Lee L (1983) Incidence of para-aortic and pelvic lymph node metastases in epithelial carcinoma of the ovary. Gynecol Oncol 16:95–100

Chorlton I (1987) Malignant lymphoma of the female genital tract and ovaries. In: Fox H (ed) Haines and Taylor obstetrical and gynaecological pathology (Vol. 2, 3rd edn) Churchill Livingstone, Edinburgh, p 737–762

Clarke-Pearson DL, Bandy LC, Dudzinski M, Heaston D, Creasman WT (1986) Computed tomography in evaluation of patients with ovarian carcinoma in complete clinical remission. JAMA 255:627–630

Coffin CM, Adcock LL, Dehner LP (1985) The second-look operation for ovarian neoplasms: a study of 85 cases emphasizing cytologic and histologic problems. Int J Gynecol Pathol 4:97–109

Cohen CJ (1985) Surgical considerations in ovarian cancer. Semin Oncol 12:53–56

Cohen CJ, Goldberg JD, Holland JF, Bruckner HW, Deppe G, Gusberg SB, Wallach RC, Kabakow B, Rodin (1983) Improved therapy with cisplatin regimens for patients with ovarian carcinoma (FIGO Stages III and IV) as measured by surgical end-staging (second look operation). Am J Obstet Gynecol 145:955–965

Colgan TJ, Norris HJ (1983) Ovarian epithelial tumors of low malignant potential: a review. Int J Gynecol Pathol 1:367–382

Copeland LJ (1985) Second-look laparotomy for ovarian carcinoma. Clin Obstet Gynecol 28:816–823

Copeland LJ, Gershenson DM (1986) Ovarian cancer recurrences in patients with no macroscopic tumor at second-look laparotomy. Obstet Gynecol 68:873–874

Creasman WT, Abu-Ghazaleh S, Schmidt HJ (1978) Retroperitoneal metastatic spread of ovarian cancer. Gynecol Oncol 6:447–449

Curry SL, Zambo MM, Nahhas WA, Jahshan AE, Whitney CW, Mortel R (1981) Second-look laparotomy for ovarian cancer. Gynecol Oncol 11:114–118

Cutler SJ, Myers MH, Green SB (1975) Trends in survival rates of patients with cancer. N Engl J Med 293:122–124

Czernobilsky B (1985) Common epithelial tumors of the ovary. In Roth LM & Czernobilsky B (eds) Tumors and tumorlike conditions of the ovary (Vol 6 Contemporary Issues in Surgical Pathology). Churchill Livingstone, New York, p 11–41

Dauplat J, Ferriere J-P, Gorbinet M, Legros M, Chollet P, Giraud B, Plagne R (1986) Second-look laparotomy in managing epithelial ovarian carcinoma. Cancer 57:1627–1631

Delclos L, Quinlan E (1969) Malignant tumors of the ovary managed with postoperative megavoltage irradiation. Radiology 93:659–663

Dienemann D, Pickartz H (1987) So-called peritoneal implants of ovarian carcinomas. Problems in differential diagnosis. Pathol Res Pract 182:195–201

DiSaia PJ, Creasman WT (1984) Clinical gynecologic oncology. The CV Mosby Company, St. Louis, p 275–278

Dyre JC (1984) Intraperitoneal pressure in the human. Surg Gynecol Obstet 87:472–475

Ehrmann RL, Federschneider JM, Knapp RC (1980) Distinguishing lymph node metastases from benign glandular inclusions in low grade ovarian carcinoma. Am J Obstet Gynecol 136:737–746

Einhorn N (1978) Acute leukemia after chemotherapy (Melphalan). Cancer 41:444–447

Farhi DC, Siverberg SG (1982) Pseudometastases in female genital cancer. Pathol Annu 17 (Pt 1):47–76

Feldman GB, Knapp RC, Arder SE, Hellman S (1972) The role of lymphatic obstruction in the formation of ascites in a murine ovarian carcinoma. Cancer Res 32:1663–1666

Feldman GB, Knapp RC (1974) Lymphatic drainage of the peritoneal cavity and its significance in ovarian cancer. Am J Obstet Gynecol 119.991–994

Fuks Z (1975) External radiotherapy of ovarian cancer. Standard approaches and new frontiers. Semin Oncol 2:253–266

Gershenson DM, Copeland LJ, Wharton JT, Atkinson EN, Sneige N, Edwards CL, Rutledge FN (1985) Prognosis of surgically determined complete responders in advanced ovarian cancer. Cancer 55:1129–1135

Goldhirsch A, Triller JK, Greiner R, Dreher E, Davis BW (1983) Computed tomography prior to second-look operation in advanced ovarian cancer. Obstet Gynecol 62:630–634

Greco FA, Julian CG, Richardson RL, Burnett L, Hande KR, Oldham RK (1981) Advanced ovarian cancer: brief intensive combination chemotherapy and second-look operation. Obstet Gynecol 58:199–205

Griffiths CT (1975) Surgical resection of tumor bulk in the primary treatment of ovarian carcinoma: Symposium on ovarian cancer. Natl Cancer Inst Monogr 42:101–104

Griffiths CT, Fuller AF Jr (1978) Intensive surgical and chemotherapeutic management of advanced ovarian cancer. Surg Clin North Am 58:131–142

Griffiths CT, Parker LM, Fuller AF Jr (1979) Role of cytoreductive surgical treatment in the management of advanced ovarian cancer. Cancer Treat Rep 63:235–240

Griffiths CT, Parker L (1986) Cancer of the ovary. In: Knapp RC, Berkowitz RS (eds) Gynecologic oncology, Macmillan, New York, p 313–375

Hacker NF, Berek JS, Lagasse LD, Nieberg RK, Elasoff RM (1983) Primary cytoreductive surgery for ovarian cancer. Obstet Gynecol 61:413–420

Hanson MB, Powell DE, Donaldson ES, Van Nagell JR Jr (1980) Treatment of epithelial ovarian carcinoma by surgical debulking followed by single alkylating agent chemotherapy. Gynecol Oncol 10:337–342

Hart WR (1981) Pathology of malignant and borderline epithelial tumors of ovary. In: Coppleson M (ed) Gynecologic oncology. Fundamental principles and clinical practice. Churchill Livingstone, Edinburgh, p 633–654

Hayes DM, Cvitkovic E, Golbey RB, Scheiner E, Helson L, Krakoff IH (1977) High-dose cis-platinumdiamminedichloride. Amelioration of renal toxicity by mannitol diuresis. Cancer 39:1372–1381

Helewa ME, Kreport GV, Lotocki R (1986) Staging laparotomy in early epithelial ovarian carcinoma. Am J Obstet Gynecol 154:282–286

Henderson C, Frei E (1979) Adriamycin and the heart. N Engl J Med 300:310–311

Heydenrych JJ, Villet WT, du Toit DF (1979) Gliomatosis peritonei: the value of a "second look" operation. J Surg Oncol 12:119–125

Higgins GM, Graham AS (1929) Lymphatic damage from the peritoneal cavity in the dog. Arch Surg 19:453–465

Ho AG, Beller U, Speyer JL, Colombo N, Wernz J, Beckman EM (1987) A reassessment of the role of second-look laparotomy in advanced ovarian cancer. J Clin Oncol 5:1316–1321

Holtz F, Hart WR (1982) Krukenberg tumors of the ovary. A clinicopathologic analysis of 27 cases. Cancer 50:2438–2447

Hopkins MP, Kumar NB, Morley GW (1987) An assessment of pathologic features and treatment modalities in ovarian tumors of low malignant potential. Obstet Gynecol 70:923–929

Hsu YK, Parmley TH, Rosenshein NB, Bhagavan BS, Woodruff JD (1980) Neoplastic and non-neoplastic mesothelial proliferations in pelvic lymph nodes. Obstet Gynecol 55:83–88

International Federation of Gynecology and Obstetrics (1982) Annual report on the results of treatment in gynecological cancer. Vol. 18. Radiumhemmet, Stockholm

Joyeux H, Szawlowski AW, Saint-Aubert B, Elazhary MM, Solassol C, Pujol H (1986) Aggressive regional surgery for advanced ovarian cancer. Cancer 57:142–147

Julian CG, Goss J, Blanchard K, Woodruff JD (1974) Biologic behavior of primary ovarian malignancy. Obstet Gynecol 44:873–884

Kapadia SB, Krause JR (1978) Ovarian carcinoma terminating in acute nonlymphocytic leukemia following alkylating agent therapy. Cancer 41:1676–1679

Keettel WC, Elkins HB (1956) Experience with radioactive colloidal gold in the treatment of ovarian carcinoma. Am J Obstet Gynecol 71:553–565

Keettel WC, Pixley EE, Buchsbaum HJ (1974) Experience with peritoneal cytology in the management of gynecologic malignancies. Am J Obstet Gynecol 120:174–178

Knapp RC, Friedman EA (1974) Aortic lymph node metastases in early ovarian cancer. Am J Obstet Gynecol 119:1013–1017

Langley FA, Fox H (1987) Ovarian tumours: classification, histogenesis and aetiology. In: Fox H (ed) Haines and Taylor obstetrical and gynaecological pathology (Vol 1, 3rd edn) Churchill Livingstone, Edinburgh, p 542–555

Lash RH, Hart WR (1987) Intestinal adenocarcinoma metastatic to the ovaries. A clinicopathologic evaluation of 22 cases. Am J Surg Pathol 11:114–121

Lindgren I, Nagy EJ, Virtaina P (1968) Drainage of radiographic contrast media from the abdominal cavity. Acta Radiol [Diagn] 7:481–488

Lingeman CH (1974) Etiology of cancer of the human ovary: a review. Natl Cancer Inst Monogr 53:1603–1618

Lurain JR (1982) Newer diagnostic approaches to the evaluation of gynecologic malignancies. Obstet Gynecol Surv 37:437–448

Lynch FW (1936) A clinical review of 110 cases of ovarian carcinoma. Am J Obstet Gynecol 32:753–772

Malkasian GD Jr, Decker DG, Webb MJ (1975) Histology of epithelial tumors of the ovary: Clinical usefulness and prognostic significance of the histologic classification and grading. Semin Oncol 2:191–201

Mamtora H, Isherwood I (1982) Computized tomography in ovarian carcinoma: patterns of disease and limitations. Clin Radiol 33:165–171

Mangioni C, Bolis G, Molteni C (1979) Indications, advantages and limits of laparoscopy in ovarian cancer. Gynecol Oncol 7:47–55

Manivel JC, Wick MR, Coffin CM, Dehner LP (1988, in press) Immunohistochemistry in the differential diagnosis in the second-look operation for ovarian carcinomas. Int J Gynecol Pathol

Mc Caughey WTE (1985) Papillary peritoneal neoplasms in females. Pathol Annu 20 (Pt 2):387–404

McGowan L, Lesher LP, Norris HJ, Barnett M (1985) Misstaging ovarian cancer. Obstet Gynecol 65:568–572

Merino MJ, Edmonds P, LiVolsi V (1985) Appendiceal carcinoma metastatic to the ovaries and mimicking primary ovarian tumours. Int J Gynecol Pathol 4:110–120

Metz SA, Sevin B, Averette H, Karnei R, Hoskins R (1981) Lymphatic metastase in apparently early carcinoma of the ovary. Gynecol Oncol 12:261–267

Meyers MA (1970) The spread and localization of acute intraperitoneal effusion. Radiology 95:547–554

Meyers MA (1973) Distribution of intra-abdominal malignant seeding: dependency on dynamics of flow of ascitic fluid. AJR 119:198–206

Michael H, Roth LM (1986) Invasive and noninvasive implants in ovarian serous tumors of low malignant potential. Cancer 57:1240–1247

Miller DS, Ballon SC, Teng NNH, Seifer DB, Soriero OM (1986) A critical reassessment of second-look laparotomy in epithelial ovarian carcinoma. Cancer 57:530–535

Moench LM (1933) A clinical study of 403 caes of adenocarcinoma of the ovary. Am J Obstet Gynecol 26:22–28

Moore GE (1980) Debunking debulking. Surg Gynecol Obstet 150:395–396

Munnell EW (1968) The changing prognosis and treatment in cancer of the ovary. Am J Obstet Gynecol 100:790–805

Munnell EW (1969) Is conservative therapy ever justified in Stage I (I-A) cancer of the ovary. Am J Obstet Gynecol 103:641–653

Musumeci R, DePalo G, Kenda R, Tesoro-Tess JD, DiRe F, Petrillo R, Rilke F (1980) Retroperitoneal metastases from ovarian carcinoma: reassessment of 356 patients studied with lymphography. AJR 134:449–452

Nelson JH (1975) Importance of maximum procedure in ovarian cancer. Natl Cancer Inst Monogr 42:109–111

Nielsen SNJ, Scheithauer BW, Gaffey TA (1985) Gliomatosis peritonei. Cancer 56:2499–2503

Nilogg JM, Bast RC, Schaetzl EM, Knapp RC (1985) Predictive value of CA 125 antigen levels in second-look procedures for ovarian cancer. Am J Obstet Gynecol 151:981–986

Norris CC, Murphy DP (1932) Malignant ovarian neoplasms. Am J Obstet Gynecol 23:833–837

Norris HJ, Zirkin HJ, Benson WL (1976) Immature (malignant) teratoma of the ovary. A clinical and pathologic study of 58 cases. Cancer 37:2359–2372

Nouwen EJ, Hendrix PG, Dauwe S, Eerdekens, MW, DeBroe ME (1987) Tumor markers in the human ovary and its neoplasms. A comparative immunohistochemical study. Am J Pathol 126:230–242

Overholt RH (1931) Intraperitoneal pressure. Arch Surg 22:691–703

Ozols RF, Young RC (1987) Ovarian cancer. Curr Probl Cancer 11:(No 2) 61–93

Parker RT, Parker CH, Wilbanks GD (1970) Cancer of the ovary: survival studied based upon operative therapy, chemotherapy and radiotherapy. Am J Obstet Gynecol 108:878–888

Perrone T, Steiner M, Dehner LP (1986) Nodal gliomatosis and -fetoprotein production. Two unusual facets of grade I ovarian teratoma. Arch Pathol Lab Med 110:975–977

Phillips BP, Buchsbaum HJ, Lifshitz S (1979) Reexploration after treatment for ovarian carcinoma. Gynecol Oncol 8:339–345

Piura B, Bar-David J, Glezerman M, Zirkin HJ (1986) Bilateral ovarian involvement as the only manifestation of malignant lymphoma. J Surg Oncol 33:126–128

Piver MS, Lele S, Barlow JJ (1976) Preoperative and intraoperative evaluation in ovarian malignancy. Obstet Gynecol 48:312–315

Piver MS, Barlow JJ, Lele SB (1978) Incidence of subclinical metastasis in Stage I and II ovarian carcinoma. Obstet Gynecol 52:100–104

Plentl AA, Friedman EA (1971) Lymphatic system of the female genitalia: the morphologic basis of oncologic diagnosis and therapy. WB Saunders, Philadelphia

Raju KS, McKenna JA, Barker GH, Wiltshaw E, Jones JM (1982) Second-look operations in the planned management of advanced ovarian carcinoma. Am J Obstet Gynecol 144:650–654

Reiner RR, Hoover R, Fraumeni JR Jr, Young RC (1977) Acute leukemia after alkylating-agent therapy of ovarian cancer. N Engl J Med 297:177–181

Richardson GS, Scully RE, Nikrui N, Nelson JH (1985) Common epithelial cancer of the ovary. N Engl J Med 312:415–424

Robboy SJ, Scully RE, Norris HJ (1974) Carcinoid metastatic to the ovary. A clinicopathologic analysis of 35 cases. Cancer 33:798–811

Robboy SJ, Norris HJ, Scully RE (1975) Insular carcinoid primary in the ovary. A clinicopathologic analysis of 48 cases. Cancer 36:404–418

Roberts WS, Hodel K, Rich WM, DiSaia PJ (1982) Second-look laparotomy in the management of gynecologic malignancy. Gynecol Oncol 13:345–355

Rosenoff SH, DeVita VT Jr, Hubbard S, Young RC (1975a) Peritoneoscopy in the staging and follow-up of ovarian cancer. Semin Oncol 2:223–228

Rosenoff SH, Young RC, Anderson T, Bagley C, Chabner B, Schein PS, Hubbard S, DeVita VT Jr (1975b) Peritoneoscopy: a valuable staging tool in ovarian carcinoma. Ann Intern Med 88:37–41

Russell P (1987) Common epithelial tumours of the ovary. In: Fox H (ed) Haines and Taylor obstetrical and gynaecological pathology (Vol 1, 3rd edn) Churchill Livingstone, Edinburgh, p 556–622

Russell P, Bannatyne PM, Solomon HJ, Stoddard LD, Tattersall MHN (1985) Multifocal tumorigenesis in the upper female genital tract – implications for staging and management. Int J Gynecol Pathol 4:192–210

Salmon SE, Hamburger AW, Soehnlein BS, Durie GM, Alberts DS, Moon TE (1978) Quantitation of differential sensitivity of human tumor stem cells to anticancer drugs. N Engl J Med 298:1321–1327

Schwartz PE, Smith JP (1980) Second-look operations in ovarian cancer. Am J Obstet Gynecol 138:1124–1130

Silva EG (1987) Gynecologic specimens. In: Silva EG & Kraemer BB (eds) Intraoperative pathologic diagnosis. Williams & Wilkins, Baltimore, p 103–110

Smith JP, Day TG Jr (1979) Review of ovarian cancer at the University of Texas Systems Cancer Center, M.D. Anderson Hospital and Tumor Institute. Am J Obstet Gynecol 135:984–993

Smith JP, Rutledge F, Wharton JT (1972) Chemotherapy of ovarian cancer. Cancer 30:1565–1571

Smith JP, Delgado G, Rutledge G (1976) Second-look operation in ovarian cancer: postchemotherapy. Cancer 38:1438–1442

Spinelli P, Luini A, Pizzetti P, De Palo GM (1976) Laparoscopy in staging and restaging of 95 patients with ovarian carcinoma. Tumori 62:493–501

Stern J, Buscema J, Rosensheim N, Siegelman S (1981) Can computed tomography substitute for second look operations in ovarian carcinoma? Gynecol Oncol 11:82–88

Stuart GLE, Jeffries M, Stuart JL, Anderson RJ (1982) The changing role of "second-look" laparotomy in the management of epithelial carcinoma of the ovary. Am J Obstet Gynecol 142:612–616

Tobias JS, Griffiths CT (1976) Management of ovarian cancer: current concepts and future prospects. N Engl J Med 294:818–823

Ulbright TM, Roth LM (1985) Secondary tumors of the ovary. In: Roth LM, Czernobilsky B (eds) Tumors and tumorlike conditions of the ovary (Vol 6, Contemporary Issues in Surgical Pathology). Churchill Livingstone, New York, pp 129–152

Walton L, Ellenberg SS, Major F Jr, Miller A, Park R, Young RC (1987) Results of second-look laparotomy in patients with early-stage ovarian carcinoma. Obstet Gynecol 70:770–773

Webb MJ, Decker DG, Mussey E, Williams TJ (1973) Factors influencing survival in Stage I ovarian cancer. Am J Obstet Gynecol 116:222–228

Webb MJ, Snyder JA Jr, Williams TJ, Decker DG (1982) Second-look laparotomy in ovarian cancer. Gynecol Oncol 14:285–293

Wharton JT, Henson J (1981) Surgery for common epithelial tumors of the ovary. Cancer 48:582–589

Wijnen JA, Rosensheim NB (1980) Surgery in ovarian cancer. Arch Surg 115:863–868

Williams TJ, Dockerty MB (1976) Status of the contralateral ovary in encapsulatet low grade malignant tumors of the ovary. Surg Gynecol Obstet 143:763–766

Wu P-C, Qu J-Y, Lang J-H, Huang R-L, Tang M-Y, Lian L-J (1986) Lymph node metastasis of ovarian cancer: a preliminary survey of 74 cases of lymphadenectomy. Am J Obstet Gynecol 155:1103–1108

Young RC (1987) A second look at second-look laparotomy. J Clin Oncol 5:1311–1313

Young RC, Chabner BA, Hubbard SP, Fisher RI, Bender RA, Anderson T, Simon RM, Canellos GP, DeVita VT (1978) Advanced ovarian adenocarcinoma. A prospective clincal trial of Melphalon (L-PAM) versus combination chemotherapy. N Engl J Med 299:1261–1266

Young RC, Decker DG, Wharton JT, Piver MS, Sindelar WF, Edwards BK, Smith JP (1983) Staging laparotomy in early ovarian cancer. JAMA 250:3072–3076

Young RH, Scully RE (1987) Metastatic tumors of the ovary. In Kurman RJ (ed) Blaustein's pathology of the female fenital tract, 3rd edn. Springer-Verlag, New York, p 742–768

Zinsser KR, Wheeler JE (1982) Endosalpingiosis in the omentum. A study of autopsy and surgical material. Am J Surg Pathol 6:109–117

Cytopathology and Fine-Needle Aspiration in Ovarian Tumours: Its Utility in Diagnosis and Management

C. NUÑEZ

1 Introduction

Malignant ovarian tumours are often at an advanced stage when initially diagnosed. Exploratory laparotomy and histological examination are the accepted approach in evaluating pelvic masses. Cytopathology has had a minor role historically in the diagnosis and management of pelvic masses of unknown aetiology. That role usually consisted of examination of ascitic fluid or fluid obtained through culdocentesis for the presence of malignant cells. The study of culdocentesis samples in asymptomatic women has been of little help in the early diagnosis of ovarian cancer (FLOYD et al. 1969; FUNKHOUSER et al. 1975; GRAHAM et al. 1964; KEETTEL et al. 1974; McGOWAN et al. 1966). Furthermore, malignant cells in culdocentesis fluid may be derived from organs other than the ovary. Other cytological techniques more useful in the diagnosis and management of ovarian tumours include peritoneal lavage at the time of laparoscopy (CREASMAN and RUTLEDGE 1971; KEETTEL et al. 1974; YOSHIMURA et al. 1984), cul-de-sac cytology after surgery for ovarian cancer (GOLDBERG et al. 1985; VENESMAA et al. 1986), and fine-needle aspiration biopsy.

Fine needle aspiration biopsy is currently accepted as an effective tool for diagnosing primary, metastatic, or recurrent malignant tumours; benign tumours; and non-neoplastic lesions in different body locations. Its application to the diagnosis of gynecological tumours, namely, the evaluation of pelvic masses, has been controversial. Some authors have advocated aspiration biopsy as a valuable tool in the diagnosis of ovarian tumours and pelvic masses (ANG-

STROM 1975; DUDKIEWICZ et al. 1977; GANJEI and NADJI 1984; GEIER et al.
1975; GEIER and STRECKER 1981; KJELLGREN et al. 1971; KJELLGREN and ANG-
STROM 1979; KJELLGREN and ANGSTROM 1982; NORDQVIST et al. 1979; SEVIN
et al. 1979; SEVIN and NADJI 1983). However, others have raised questions about
the justification for aspirating pelvic masses, the main objection being the risk
of spilling the tumour contents into the peritoneal cavity (CHRISTOPHERSON 1983;
HAJDU and MELAMED 1984).

Spilling tumour contents into the pelvis is a valid concern when using aspiration biopsies on cystic or semicystic pelvic tumours. Therefore, it appears judi-
cious to avoid aspirating such lesions, especially early stage I and II neoplasms
in which peritoneal seeding may alter the prognosis. These lesions are better
evaluated by conventional exploratory laparotomy, where rupture and seeding
may be more easily avoided.

Advanced stage III and IV neoplasms are usually treated by reductive surgery and chemotherapy. However, selected patients with unresectable lesions
or poor surgical candidates may benefit from aspiration biopsy and avoid
further surgery when confirmation of a malignant process is required.

Fine-needle aspiration is most useful in the follow-up of patients with a
history of ovarian malignancy in which a pelvic or extrapelvic recurrence is
suspected (BELINSON et al. 1981; BONFIGLIO et al. 1979; DUNNICK et al. 1980;
FLINT et al. 1982; FORTIER et al. 1985; LARSEN et al. 1985; MORIARTY et al.
1986). In this group of patients, aspiration biopsy may obviate the need for
surgery, with its associated morbidity, and reduce the hospital cost.

2 Specimen Collection Techniques

In fine-needle aspiration biopsy, cell groups and minute tissue fragments are
removed by thin needles with an external diameter of about 0.6 mm. Because
of the thin caliber of the needle, morbidity or complications related to the
procedure are negligible (BELINSON et al. 1981; FLINT et al. 1982; GANJEI and
NADJI 1984; GEIGER and STRECKER 1981; KJELLGREN and ANGSTROM 1979;
KOVACIC et al. 1979). The equipment required usually includes a 20 ml syringe,
thin needles of different lengths, and a Franzen guide for transvaginal and
transrectal aspirations.

Many pelvic and parametrial lesions may be approached through the vagina
or the rectum. The transvaginal route is generally favored since the vagina
can be cleansed thoroughly before puncture. Transrectal aspirations carry a
higher risk of pelvic infection (GEIGER and STRECKER 1981; KJELLGREN and
ANGSTROM 1982). Most transvaginal and transrectal aspirations are performed
during examination of the patient under general anesthesia.

Nonpalpable intrapelvic masses, intra-abdominal and intrathroracic suspected metastases, and pelvic and para-aortic lymph nodes may be aspirated
after being localized by such radiologic techniques as biplanar fluoroscopy (BON-
FIGLIO et al. 1979; DUNNICK et al. 1980; KARLSSON and PERSSON 1979), ultrasonography (BELINSON et al. 1981; CRESPIGNY et al. 1985; LARSEN et al. 1985), and

computed tomography (JAQUES et al. 1978; FORTIER et al. 1985; MORIARTY et al. 1986). Laparoscopy is another useful route for aspiration of pelvic lesions encountered during laparoscopic examination (KOVACIC et al. 1979; KOVACIC et al. 1982).

Once the needle is placed within the lesion, continuous suction is applied while the needle is moved slightly back and forth. When the aspiration is accomplished, the pressure within the syringe is released and the needle is then withdrawn. The aspirated material is smeared on glass slides, which are immediately fixed in 95% ethyl, methyl, or isopropyl alcohol, or sprayed-fixed and subsequently stained by the Papanicolaou method. Conversely, the smears can be air-dried and stained with May-Grunwald-Giemsa, modified Wright-Giemsa, or haematoxylin-eosin (FRABLE 1983). In selected cases, microbacteriological, ultrastructural, and immunocytochemical studies can be performed on aspirates.

Peritoneal lavage is performed by instilling 100 to 150 ml of saline into the lower abdomen and allowing it to collect within the pelvic cavity. The fluid is then removed and processed like any other fluid sample for cytological analysis. Selected areas of the peritoneum can be sampled by irrigation with saline (CREASMAN and RUTLEDGE 1971; KEETTEL et al. 1974). Any fluid found when the peritoneal cavity is opened is also sent for analysis.

Culdocentesis samples are obtained by aspirating the culde-sac transvaginally. If no fluid is present, 10 to 20 ml of saline is injected, reaspirated, and analyzed for the presence of malignant cells (GOLDBERG et al. 1985; KEETTEL et al. 1974; VENESMAA et al. 1986).

3 Benign Lesions

Included in this group are inflammatory lesions, endometriosis, benign epithelial ovarian tumours, non-neoplastic ovarian cysts, and benign tumours arising in the broad ligament, which may simulate ovarian neoplasms.

3.1 Inflammatory Lesions

Tubo-ovarian or pelvic abcesses are usually diagnosed clinically and are seldom the target of aspiration biopsy. Aspirates from inflammatory lesions are characterized by acute inflammatory exudate, macrophages, and necrotic debris. Specific organisms may be identified (LININGER and FRABLE 1984). If infection is suspected, appropriate samples must be sent for microbiologic studies.

3.2 Endometriosis

Suspected endometriotic lesions are frequently aspirated during laparoscopy. The most common cytological presentation of endometriosis consists of macrophages laden with haemosiderin in a background of broken-down red blood

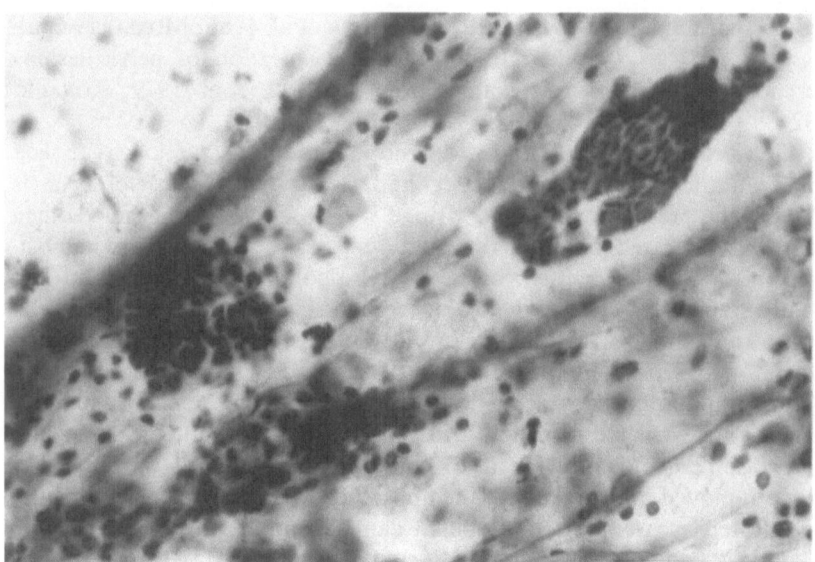

Fig. 1. Endometriosis. Degenerated endometrial cells, histiocytes and blood. Papanicolaou, × 384

cells. Endometrial cells are seldom seen or, if present, are markedly degenerated (Fig. 1). However, a diagnosis of endometriosis can be made only when endometrial cells are identified (KOVACIC et al. 1979; KOVACIC et al. 1982; NADJI et al. 1979; RAMZY et al. 1979; SEVIN and NADJI 1983).

Endometrial cells usually occur in dense aggregates. They are small, with scant, finely vacuolated cytoplasm. The nuclei are uniform, round to oval, with granular chromatin and inconspicuous nucleoli.

3.3 Non-Neoplastic Cysts

This group of lesions is usually aspirated during laparoscopy or laparotomy in patients evaluated for infertility, pelvic pain, or suspected endometriosis.

Non-neoplastic cystic lesions of the ovary include follicular and corpus luteum cysts and germinal inclusion cysts. Aspirates from these cysts usually yield sparsely cellular clear fluid containing macrophages. Due to the absence of specific cytological features, these lesions are classified as benign cysts. (KOVACIC et al. 1979, 1982; RAMZY et al. 1979). Occasionally, aspirates from corpus luteum cysts may have luteinized cells with abundant granular or finely vacuolated cytoplasms (Fig. 2). The aspirate from a haemorrhagic corpus luteum may be difficult to distinguish from endometriosis.

Aspirates from developing follicles or cysts in polycystic ovaries may have abundant cells occurring singly or in aggregates. Granulosa cells are round, with finely vacuolated cytoplasm and centrally placed nuclei with granular chromatin. Mitotic figures may be numerous. Because of the unusual abundant cellularity and mitotic figures, these aspirates can be misinterpreted as malignant (Fig. 3).

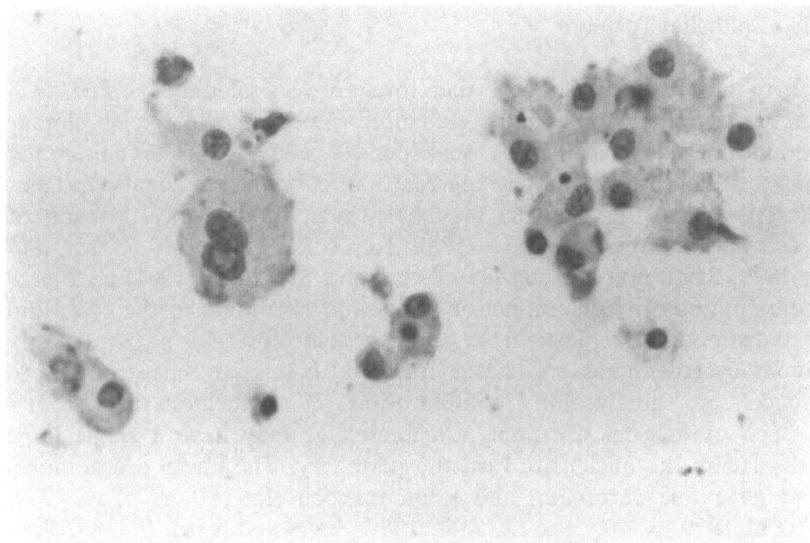

Fig. 2. Corpus luteum cyst. Groups of luteinized cells with abundant granular cytoplasm. Papanicolaou, × 384

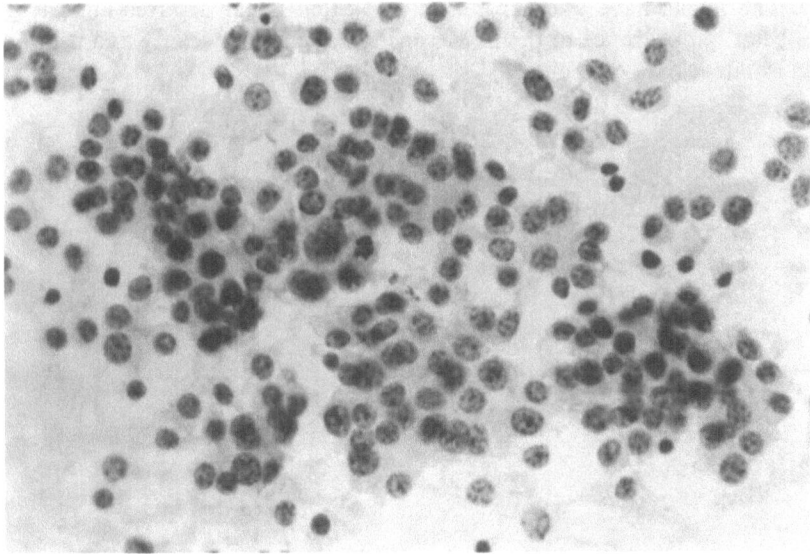

Fig. 3. Follicular cyst. Granulosa cells with coarse chromatin, and small nucleoli. A mitotic figure is seen at the center. Papanicolaou, × 384

Benign cystic lesions occurring outside the ovary, such as paratubal and paraovarian cysts, have the same cytological appearance in aspirates as non-neoplastic ovarian cysts. Aspirates yield sparsely cellular fluid containing macrophages and occasional degenerated epithelial cells.

3.4 Benign Epithelial Tumours

Most of these tumours are cystic and, therefore, are very seldom aspirated.

Benign serous cystadenomas and cystadenofibromas are cytologically similar to non-neoplastic cysts. Usually they yield sparsely cellular aspirates containing macrophages and occasionally a few aggregates of cuboidal epithelial cells lacking atypical features (Fig. 4). Cilia may be present in the apical portion of the cells (KJELLGREN and ANGSTROM 1982, KOVACIC et al. 1979; RAMZY and DELANEY 1979, SEVIN and NADJI 1983). GEIER and STRECKER (1981) have proposed radioimmunoassay determination of steroid hormones in the cyst fluid as a way to distinguish neoplastic from non-neoplastic cysts.

Mucinous cystadenomas are characterized by columnar cells arranged in "picket-fence" or "honeycomb" configurations in a mucinous background (Fig. 5). Their cytoplasms are finely vacuolated or may have a single large vacuole displacing the nucleus toward the periphery. The nuclei are homogeneous and have fine chromatin and small nucleoli (KJELLGREN et al. 1979; KOVACIC et al. 1979; RAMZY and DELANEY 1979; SEVIN and NADJI 1983). Colonic mucosal cells may contaminate transrectal aspirates and may simulate mucinous cystadenoma.

Aspirates from Brenner's tumours may contain both epithelial and mesenchymal cells. Epithelial cells are cuboidal to polygonal and occur in sheets or singly. The nuclei have fine chromatin and often linear grooves imparting a "coffee bean" appearance to them. Mesenchymal cells are scanty and usually appear as isolated, bare oval nuclei.

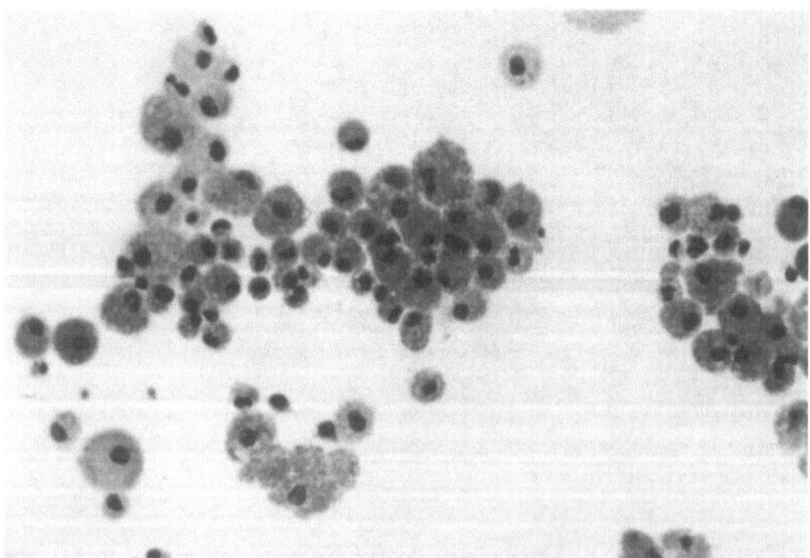

Fig. 4. Benign serous cystadenoma. Macrophages are the predominant cell type present in these benign cysts. Papanicolaou, × 192

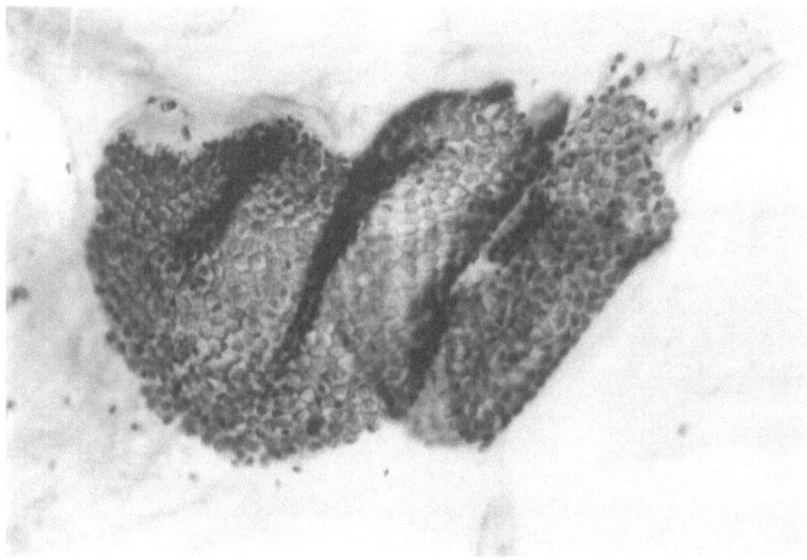

Fig. 5. Benign mucinous cystadenoma. Sheet of columnar, mucin-secreting cells in a "honey-comb" arrangement. Papanicolaou, × 192

Amorphous, eosinophilic round bodies may be seen at the center of epithelial groups or in the background (KJELLGREN and ANGSTROM 1979; RAMZY and DELANEY 1979; SEVIN and NADJI 1983).

3.5 Other Benign Lesions

Subserosal uterine myomas or myomas arising in the broad ligament may simulate ovarian tumours and be subjected to aspiration biopsy. Leiomyomas yield few or no cells on aspiration biopsy. When cells are present, they occur isolated or in small, tight bundles. The cells are elongate, have eosinophilic cytoplasms, and elongate nuclei with blunt ends (NADJI et al. 1979; SEVIN and NADJI 1983).

4 Tumours of Borderline Malignancy

This group of epithelial tumours is characterized by moderate to marked epithelial proliferation, evidenced by cellular stratification and the formation of small, solid epithelial buds. Varying degrees of nuclear atypia may be present. The only feature distinguishing these tumours from carcinomas is the absence of invasion. Since the presence or absence of invasion cannot be visualized cytologically, borderline tumours cannot be diagnosed by needle aspiration (GANJEI and NADJI 1984; KJELLGREN and ANGSTROM 1979).

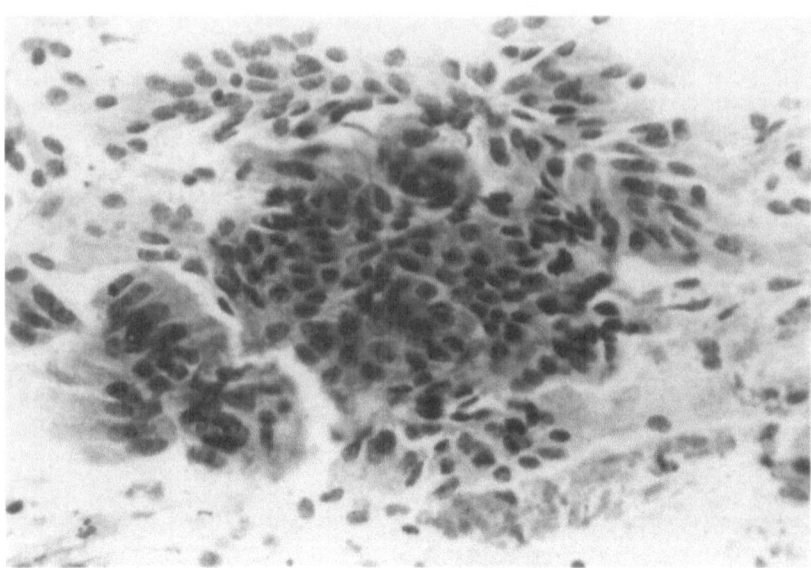

Fig. 6. Mucinous tumour of low malignant potential (borderline). Numerous endocervical-like columnar cells with slight nuclear atypicality. Necrotic debris are present in the background. Papanicolaou, × 240

Cytologically, borderline tumours present with abundant cellularity, unlike the benign epithelial lesions. The cells may occur singly or, more frequently, in groups with papillary or sheet-like configurations. Serous tumours yield cuboidal to columnar cells in papillary formations. Psammoma bodies may be present. Mucinous tumours have columnar cells with vacuolated cytoplasms in a mucinous background. Nuclear atypia is variable. Most borderline tumours are cytologically classified as carcinomas. However, occasional cases with slight degrees of cellular atypia and few cells in the aspirate may be difficult to differentiate from their benign counterparts (Fig. 6).

5 Malignant Epithelial Tumours

Needle aspirates from primary, recurrent, or metastatic malignant epithelial ovarian tumours are not diagnostic problems and, in most instances, can be recognized easily as carcinomas.

Providing a good sample is obtained, the aspirates have, in general, the features of adenocarcinomas. It is more difficult, however, to subclassify the tumours as to cell type. Serous carcinomas are difficult to distinguish from endometrioid carcinomas. Moreover, radiation may modify the cytology of the tumours, making their classification difficult (ANGSTROM 1975; GEIER et al. 1975; KJELLGREN and ANGSTROM 1979; KJELLGREN and ANGSTROM 1982; NADJI et al. 1979; RAMZY and DELANEY 1979; SEVIN and NADJI 1983).

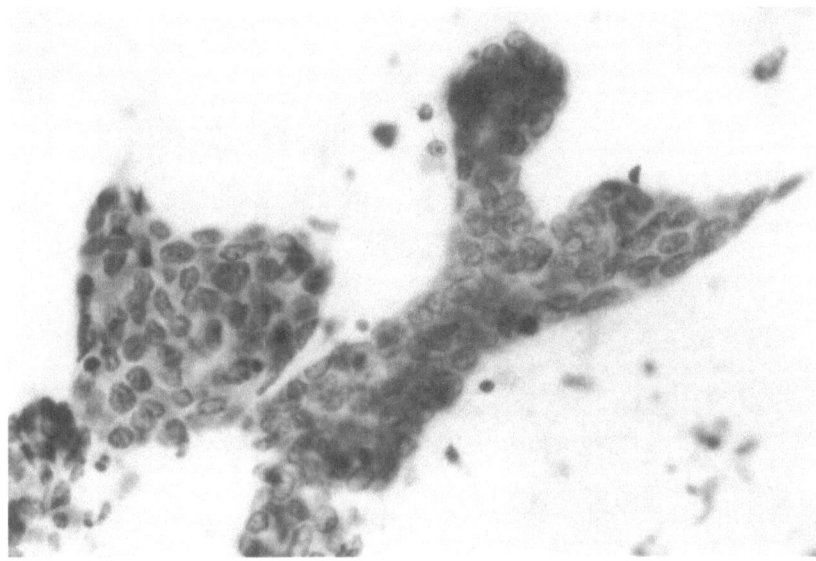

Fig. 7. Serous cystadenocarcinoma. Irregular, branching cellular groups with syncytium-like or papillary configurations. Papanicolaou, × 384

Some tumours may have differentiating features that allow them to be placed in a specific group. Serous carcinoma is characterized by cells arranged in branching papillary groups. The cells are cuboidal to low columnar, with moderate amounts of homogeneous cytoplasms. The nuclei are irregular, hyperchromatic, and have prominent nucleoli (Fig. 7) Psammoma bodies are present in about on third of these tumours but are infrequently seen in aspirates. Moreover, psammoma bodies may be seen in benign conditions, such as endosalpingosis, and therefore they are not pathognomonic of serous carcinoma.

Mucinous cystadenocarcinomas have numerous columnar cells in pools of mucin. The cells occur isolated, in clusters, and in well differentiated tumours in "picket-fence" or "honey-comb" arrangements. Their cytoplasms are abundant with single or multiple vacuoles. Nuclei are eccentrically placed and are often indented by vacuoles (Fig. 8). Mucin secreting metastatic tumours to the ovary may have a similar appearance.

Clear cell carcinoma has cells with abundant, pale staining, granular, and often vacuolated cytoplasms (Fig. 9).

Mixed adenosquamous carcinoma may arise in the ovary. The aspirates, in some instances, have both adenocarcinoma and squamous cell carcinoma components, occurring separately or, more infrequently, in continuity with one another.

Malignant mixed mullerian tumours are composed of malignant epithelial and mesenchymal elements. Aspirates from these tumours yield mostly the malignant epithelial component, which is usually a high grade carcinoma. The sarcomatous component, when present, appears as isolated for loosely cohesive

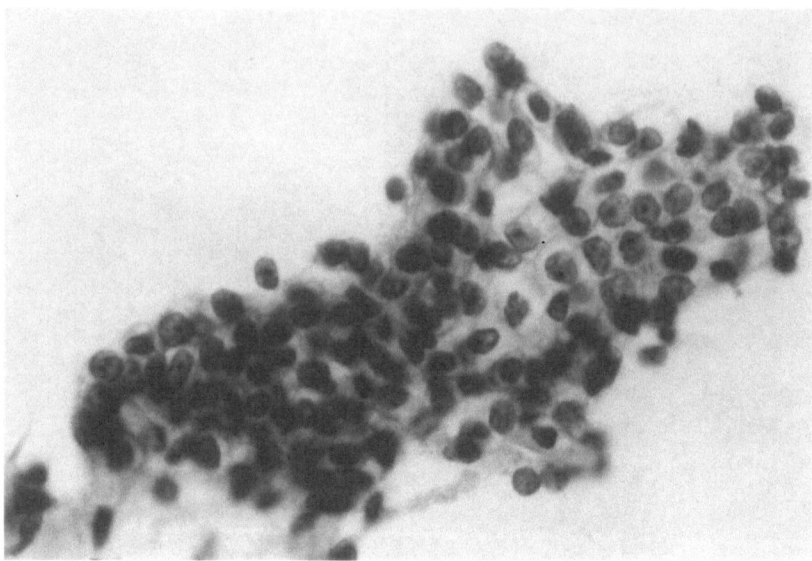

Fig. 8. Mucinous cystadenocarcinoma. Sheet of abnormal cells retaining to some extent a "honeycomb" appearance. The cytoplasm is vacuolated. The nuclei are enlarged, and have nucleoli. Papanicolaou, × 384

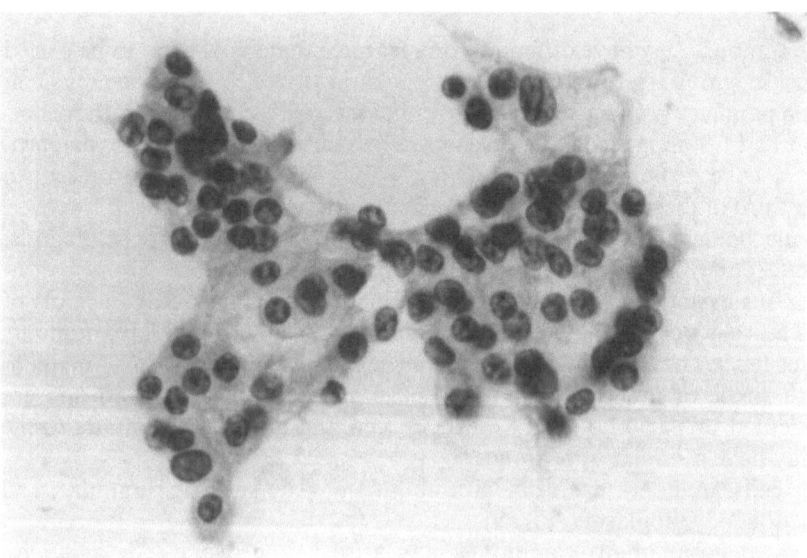

Fig. 9. Clear cell carcinoma. Group of atypical cells with a syncytium-like configuration. The cytoplasm is abundant, pale staining, and granular or finely vacuolated. Papanicolaou, × 384

abnormal spindle cells. Single, pleomorphic large cells with markedly abnormal nuclei may also be seen.

Poorly differentiated carcinomas are characterized by markedly abnormal cells with pleomorphic nuclei and scanty cytoplasms. The cells are mostly isolated or in syncytium-like aggregates among necrotic debris. Occasionally, distinction from lymphoma or sarcoma may be difficult.

6 Germ Cell Tumours and Sex-Cord Stromal Tumours

Aspiration biopsy experience with these lesions appears to be limited, judging by the few reports in the literature (BJERSING et al. 1973; EHYA and LANG 1986; FIDLER 1982; GANJEI and NADJI 1984; KJELLGREN and ANGSTROM 1979, 1982; RAMZY and DELANEY 1977; RAMZY et al. 1979; SEVIN and NADJI 1983).

Benign cystic teratoma (dermoid cyst) yields numerous anucleated squamous cells, superficial squamous cells, and abundant keratin debris. Other epithelial components such as glandular, respiratory, and intestinal epithelium may be present. However, mesenchymal components are seldom identified. Vaginal squamous cells contaminating transvaginal aspirates may be a pitfall in the diagnosis of dermoid cyst.

Dysgerminoma in aspiration biopsy is characterized by numerous, poorly cohesive cells with small amounts of cytoplasm and indistinct boundaries. The nuclei are large with clumped chromatin and large nucleoli (Fig. 10). Numerous mature lymphocytes and occasional multinucleated giant cells are sprinkled throughout the tumour. Large cell lymphoma may simulate the cytological appearance of dysgerminoma.

Immunostaining for placental alkaline phosphatase is positive in germ cell tumour and may be of value in diagnosing dysgerminoma (MANIVEL et al. 1987).

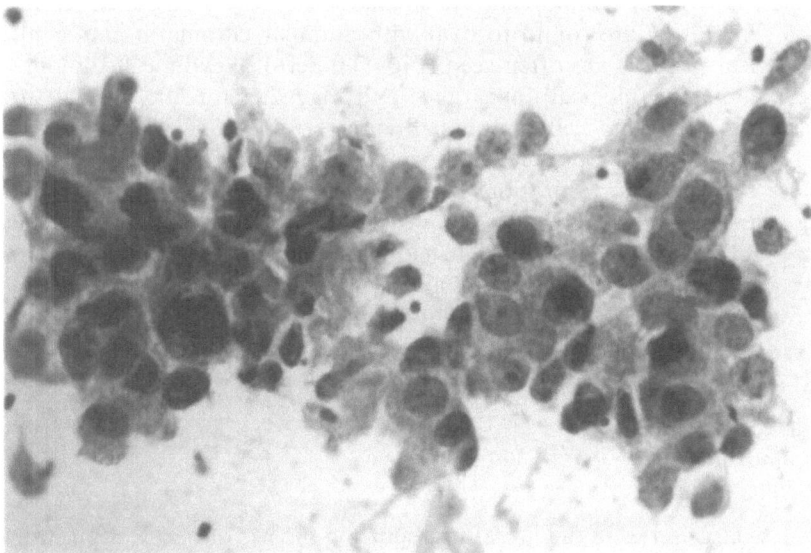

Fig. 10. Dysgerminoma. Aggregate of markedly atypical cells with large nuclei and prominent nucleoli. The cytoplasm is scanty, and the cell boundaries poorly defined. Hematoxylin-eosin, × 384

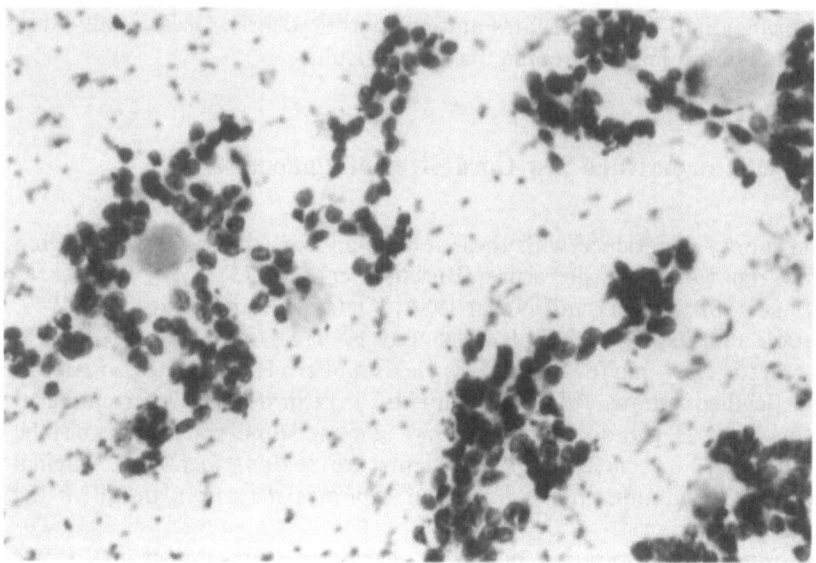

Fig. 11. Granulosa cell tumour. Acinus-like structures and thin trabeculae made up of small cells with hyperchromatic nuclei. The amorphus, round globules within the acinus-like structures correspond to Call-Exners bodies. Nuclear grooves are also present. Papanicolaou, × 240

Granulosa cell tumours present with many cells arranged singly, in compact groups, or in trabeculae. Some have small, acinus-like structures with a central mass of amorphous eosinophilic material. These structures correspond to Call-Exner bodies. Individual tumour cells are small and homogeneous, with scanty cytoplasms. The nuclei are round to oval with granular chromatin and small nucleoli. Nuclear grooves are often seen (Fig. 11). Sertoli-Leydig cell tumours may have a similar cytological appearance and may therefore be difficult to distinguish from granulosa cell tumours. Brenner's tumours, with prominent nuclear grooves and hyalin globules, also simulate the cytological presentation of granulosa cell tumours. Aspirations from neoplasms in the fibroma-thecoma group are sparsely cellular. They are composed of isolated or bundled spindle cells with scanty cytoplasm and oval to elongate nuclei with fine chromatin. In some cases, luteinized cells with more abundant, finely vacuolated cytoplasm may be present. Aspirates from these tumours can be misinterpreted as leiomyomas.

7 Clinicopathological Correlation

There are few large series in the literature reporting the use of needle aspiration biopsy to diagnose ovarian tumours (DUDKIEWICZ et al. 1977; GEIER and STRECKER 1981; KJELLGREN et al. 1971; KJELLGREN and ANGSTROM 1979, 1982).

Other series report the use of aspiration biopsy in the diagnosis or follow-up of patients with gynecological malignancies, including ovarian tumours (BELINSON et al. 1981; BONFIGLIO et al. 1979; CRESPIGNY et al. 1985; FLINT et al. 1982; FORTIER et al. 1985; MORIARTY et al. 1986; NORDQVIST et al. 1979; SEVIN et al. 1979).

Fine-needle aspiration biopsy can differentiate between benign and malignant ovarian tumours with great accuracy. Furthermore, in many instances, it is also possible to classify the tumour correctly. KJELLGREN and ANGSTROM (1982) reported a series of 236 ovarian tumours subjected to fine-needle aspiration biopsy. The overall diagnostic accuracy was 86% for malignant tumours and 91% for benign lesions. There were no false negatives; however, four false positive cases were encountered. Seventeen cases were reported as suspicious for malignancy. Of those, six were benign, nine were malignant, and two were still inconclusive on follow-up. GEIGER and STRECKER (1981) reported similar figures with an overall accuracy of 76% for malignant tumours and 91% for benign lesions. They had no false positive cases. However, they had 11.3% false negatives.

Other series describing the results of needle aspiration in patients with primary, recurrent, or metastatic pelvic or extrapelvic lesions report a reliability of 90% or better in distinguishing benign from malignant lesions (BELINSON et al. 1981; FORTIER et al. 1985; MORIARTY et al. 1986; SEVIN et al. 1979). The number of false positive diagnoses in these series varies from none to 3.5%. By applying strict cytopathological criteria of malignancy the false positive rate should be kept at zero.

Almost all series have a number of false negatives, which may be as high as 25% of the cases. Therefore, no major therapeutic descisions should be based on a negative result. If there is strong clinical suspicion of malignancy despite a negative aspiration biopsy, a second aspiration biopsy or open biopsy have to be considered.

Some of the most frequent causes of false negative diagnoses are failure to needle the lesion, small size of the lesion, previous radiation therapy with the subsequent fibrosis, and attempts to interpret suboptimal specimens. By selecting patients carefully and using a team approach, with a physician proficient in the technique of needle biopsy and a pathologist familar with the interpretation of the aspirate, results can be significantly improved and false negative and unsatisfactory rates reduced. Knowing the patient's age, clinical history, location of the lesion, and histopathologic features of ovarian neoplasms is also of utmost importance.

Despite its limitations in the diagnosis and management of ovarian tumours, cytology may be successfully used in the following clinical situations: 1) diagnosis of primary, high stage pelvic masses in patients in whom exploratory laparotomy is not feasible; 2) follow-up of patients with known ovarian tumours in whom pelvic or extrapelvic recurrences or metastases are suspected; 3) evaluation of benign pelvic lesions during laparoscopy; 4) peritoneal lavage and cul-de-sac cytology in the evaluation and staging of patients with ovarian neoplasms. In most of these instances, fine-needle aspiration biopsy offers an accurate, relatively inexpensive, and virtually complicationfree alternative to surgery.

The presence of malignant cells in peritoneal fluid or fluid collected by peritoneal lavage at the time of laparotomy indicates a poor prognosis (CREAS-MAN and RUTLEDGE 1971; KEETTEL et al. 1974). Especially important are patients with FIGO stages I and II in whom the presence of malignant cells (subgroup C) may have an influence in prognosis and in the administration of intraperitoneal radioactive compounds (YOSHIMURA et al. 1984).

Cul-de-sac cytology may be of additional help in the follow-up of patients treated for ovarian cancer in whom residual disease or pelvic recurrences are suspected (GOLDBERG et al. 1985; VENESMAA et al. 1986).

References

Angstrom T (1975) Fine-needle aspiration biopsy in diagnosis and classification of ovarian tumors. In: DeWatteville H (ed) Diagnosis and treatment of ovarian neoplastic alterations. Excerpta Medica, Basel, pp 67–72

Belinson JL, Lynn JM, Papillo JL, Lee K, Korson R (1981) Fine-needle aspiration cytology in the management of gynecologic cancer. Am J Obstet Gynecol 139:148–153

Bjersing L, Frankendal B, Angstrom T (1973) Studies on a feminizing ovarian mesenchymoma (granulosa cell tumor). I. Aspiration biopsy cytology, histology, and ultrastructure. Cancer 32:1360–1369

Bonfiglio TA, MacIntosh PK, Patten SF, Cafer DJ, Woodworth FE, Kim CW (1979) Fine needle aspiration cytopathology of retroperitoneal lymph nodes in the evaluation of metastatic disease. Acta Cytol 23:126–130

Christopherson WW (1983) Cytologic detection and diagnosis of cancer: its contributions and limitations. Cancer 51:1201–1208

Creasman WT, Rutledge F (1971) The prognostic value of peritoneal cytology in gynecologic malignant disease. Am J Obstet Gynecol 110:773–781

Crespigny LC, Robinson HP, Davoren RAM, Fortune DW (1985) Ultrasound-guided puncture for gynecological and pelvic lesions. Aust NZ, J Obstet Gynecol 25:227–229

Dudkiewicz J, Biniszkiewicz W, Blecharz A (1977) The value of fine needle biopsy in the diagnosis of ovarian tumors in women. Arch Geschwülstforsch 47:450–454

Dunnick NR, Fisher RI, Chu EW, Young RC (1980) Percutaneous aspiration of retroperitoneal lymph nodes in ovarian cancer. AJR 135:109–113

Ehya M, Lang WR (1986) Cytology of granulosa cell tumor of the ovary. Am J Clin Pathol 85:402–405

Fidler WJ (1982) Recurrent granulosa-cell tumor. Aspiration cytology findings. Acta Cytol 26:688–690

Flint A, Terhart K, Murad TM, Taylor PT (1982) Confirmation of metastases by fine needle aspiration biopsy in patients with gynecologic malignancies. Gynecol Oncol 14:382–391

Floyd WS, Boyce CR, Goodman P, Mandell G, Evans TN (1969) Peritoneal lavage and filtration for cytology. Am J Obstet Gynecol 103:425–429

Fortier KJ, Clarke-Pearson DL, Creasman WT, Johnston WW (1985) Fine-needle aspiration in gynecology: Evaluation of extrapelvic lesions in patients with gynecologic malignancy. Obstet Gynecol 65:67–72

Frable WJ (1983) Thin-needle aspiration biopsy. WB Saunders, Philadelphia, pp 17–19

Funkhouser JW, Hunter KK, Thompson NJ (1975) The diagnostic value of cul-de-sac aspiration in the detection of ovarian carcinoma. Acta Cytol 19:538–541

Ganjei P, Nadji M (1984) Aspiration cytology of ovarian neoplasms. A review. Acta Cytol 28:329–332

Geier GR, Kraus H, Schuhmann R (1975) Fine-needle aspiration biopsy in ovarian tumors. In: DeWatterville H (ed) Diagnosis and treatment of ovarian neoplastic alterations. Excerpta Medica, Basel, pp 73–76

Geiger GR, Strecker JR (1981) Aspiration cytology and E2 content in ovarian tumors. Acta Cytol 25:400–406

Goldberg G, Learmonth G, Bloch B, Levin W (1985) Role of cul-de-sac aspiration cytology in the management and follow up of patients with ovarian carcinoma. A preliminary report. J Reprod Med 30:867–870

Graham JB, Graham RM, Schueller EF (1964) Preclinical detection of ovarian cancer. Cancer 17:1414–1432

Hajdu SI, Melamed MR (1984) Limitations of aspiration cytology in the diagnosis of primary neoplasms. Acta Cytol 28:337–354

Jaques PF, Staab E, Richey W, Photopulos G, Swanton M (1978) CT-assisted pelvic and abdominal aspiration biopsies in gynecologic malignancies. Radiology 128:651–655

Karlsson S, Persson PH (1979) Angiography, ultrasound and fine-needle aspiration biopsy in the evaluation of gynecologic tumors. Acta Radiol [Diagn] 20:779–788

Keettel WC, Pixley EA, Buchsbaum HJ (1974) Experience with peritoneal cytology in the management of gynecologic malignancies. Am J Obstet Gynecol 120:174–182

Kjellgren O, Angstrom T, Bergman F, Wiklund DE (1971) Fine-needle aspiration biopsy in diagnosis and classification of ovarian carcinoma. Cancer 28:967–976

Kjellgren O, Angstrom T (1979) Transvaginal and transrectal aspiration biopsy in diagnosis and classification of ovarian tumors in: Zajicek J (ed) Aspiration biopsy cytology, part 2, Cytology of infradiaphragmatic organs. S Karger, Basel, pp 80–103

Kjellgren O, Angstrom T (1982) Aspiration biopsy cytology of ovarian tumors. In: Blaustein A (ed) Pathology of the female genital tract, 2nd edn. Springer-Verlag, New York, pp 741–751

Kovacic J, Rainer S, Levicnik, Cizelj T (1979) Cytology of benign ovarian lesions in connection with laparoscopy. In: Zajicek J (ed) Aspiration biopsy cytology, part 2, Cytology of infradiaphragmatic organs. S Karger, Basel, pp 57–79

Kovacic J, Rainer S, Levicnik A (1982) Aspiration cytology of normal structures and non-neoplastic cysts of the ovary. In: Blaustein A (ed) Pathology of the female genital tract, 2nd edn. Springer-Verlag, New York, pp 716–740

Larsen T, Torp-Pedersen S, Bostofte E, Rank F (1985) Transperineal fine needle biopsy of gynecological tumors guided by transrectal ultrasound: A new method. Gynecol Oncol 22:281–287

Lininger JR, Frable WJ (1984) Diagnosis of actinomycosis by fine needle aspiration. A case report. Acta Cytol 28:601–604

Manivel JC, Jessurun J, Wick MR, Dehner LP (1987) Placental alkaline phosphatase immunoreactivity in testicular germ-cell neoplasms. Am J Surg Pathol 11:21–29

McGowan L, Stein DB, Miller W (1966) Cul-de-sac aspiration for diagnostic cytologic study. Am J Obstet Gynecol 96:413–417

Moriarty AT, Glant MD, Stehman FB (1986) The role of fine needle aspiration cytology in the management of gynecologic malignancies. Acta Cytol 30:59–64

Nadji M, Greening SE, Sevin BU, Averette HE, Nordqvist SRB, Ng ABP (1979) Fine needle aspiration cytology in gynecologic onocology II. Morphologic aspects. Acta Cytol 23:380–388

Nordqvist SRB, Sevin BU, Nadji M, Greening S, Ng ABP (1979) Fine needle aspiration cytology in gynecologic oncology. I. Diagnostic accuracy. Obstet Gynecol 54:719–724

Ramzy I, Delaney M (1977) Signet-ring cell stromal tumor of ovary. Cytologic appearances of fine needle aspiration biopsy. Acta Cytol 21:14–17

Ramzy I, Delaney M (1979) Fine needle aspiration of ovarian masses. I. Correlative cytologic and histologic study of celomic epithelial neoplasms. Acta Cytol 23:97–104

Ramzy I, Delaney M, Rose P (1979) Fine needle aspiration of ovarian masses. II. Correlative cytologic and histologic study of non-neoplastic cysts and noncelomic epithelial neoplasms. Acta Cytol 23:185–193

Sevin BU, Greening SE, Nadji M, Ng ABP, Averette HE, Nordqvist SRB (1979) Fine needle aspiration cytology in gynecologic oncology. I. Clinical aspects. Acta Cytol 23:277–281

Sevin BU, Nadji M (1983) Pelvic fine needle aspiration cytology in gynecology. In: Linsk JA, Franzen S (eds) Clinical aspiration cytology. JB Lippincott, Philadelphia, pp 221–242

Venesmaa P, Vesterinen E, Kivisaari L, Nieminen U (1986) Pervaginal cul-de-sac cytology and CT in the follow up care of patients with advanced ovarian cancer. Gynecol Oncol 25:84–88

Yoshimura S, Scully RE, Taft PD, Herrington JB (1984) Peritoneal fluid cytology in patients with ovarian cancer. Obstet Gynecol 17:161–167

Prognostic Significance of Pathologic Features of Ovarian Carcinoma

S.G. Silverberg

Introduction

The subject of the relationship of histologic features to prognosis and treatment in ovarian cancer is obviously a broad one, considering the many histologic types of ovarian that exist, not to mention the rapidly changing therapeutic strategies that have evolved within the past decade. Since the great majority of primary malignant tumors of the ovary are of "common epithelial" type (those thought to arise ultimately from the mesothelium covering the ovarian surface) – over 90% in the population-based series of KATSUBE et al. (1982) – my comments in this chapter will be confined to this group of tumors.

1 World Health Organization Classification and Nomenclature of "Common Epithelial" Tumors of the Ovary

The World Health Organization (WHO) Classification of Ovarian Tumors was published in 1973 (SEROV et al. 1973), after ten years of deliberation by a committee composed of representatives of seven nations. The genesis of this classification has been discussed in detail by SCULLY (1975). It is reproduced in Table 1, since it represents the classification system that is almost universally utilized today.

Table 1. Who histologic classification of ovarian tumors: common "epithelial" tumors

I. Serous tumors

A. Benign
    1. Cystadenoma and papillary cystadenoma
    2. Surface papilloma
    3. Adenofibroma and cystadenofibroma

B. Of borderline malignancy (carcinomas of low malignant potential)
    1. Cystadenoma and papillary cystadenoma
    2. Surface papilloma
    3. Adenofibroma and cystadenofibroma

C. Malignant
    1. Adenocarcinoma, papillary adenocarcinoma,
      and papillary cystadenocarcinoma
    2. Surface papillary carcinoma
    3. Malignant adenofibroma and cystadenofibroma

II. Mucinous tumors

A. Benign
    1. Cystadenoma
    2. Adenofibroma and cystadenofibroma

B. Of borderline malignancy (carcinomas of low malignant potential)
    1. Cystadenoma
    2. Adenofibroma and cystadenofibroma

C. Malignant
    1. Adenocarcinoma and cystadenocarcinoma
    2. Malignant adenofibroma and cystadenofibroma

III. Endometrioid tumors

A Benign
    1. Adenoma and cystadenoma
    2. Adenofibroma and cystadenofibroma

B. Of borderline malignancy (carcinomas of low malignant potential)
    1. Adenoma and cystadenoma
    2. Adenofibroma and cystadenofibroma

C. Malignant
    1. Carcinoma
      a) Adenocarcinoma
      b) Adenoacanthoma
      c) Malignant adenofibroma and cystadenofibroma
    2. Endometrioid stromal sarcomas
    3. Mesodermal (Mullerian) mixed tumors, homologous and heterologous

IV. Clear cell (mesonephroid) tumors

A. Benign: adenofibroma

B. Of borderline malignancy (carcinomas of low malignant potential)

C. Malignant: carcinoma

V. Brenner tumors

A. Benign

B. Of borderline malignancy (proliferating)

C. Malignant

Table 1 (continued)

VI. Mixed epithelial tumors

A. Benign

B. Of borderline malignancy

C. Malignant

VII. Undifferentiated carcinoma

VIII. Unclassified epithelial tumors

---

2 "Borderline" Tumors

One of the most important features of the WHO classification – and of its precursor classification by the International Federation of Gynaecology and Obstetrics (SCULLY 1975) – was its recognition of a group of tumors that were classified as "of borderline malignancy (carcinomas of low malignant potential)". [1] These tumors, which had been recognized for many years previously by some but not all authors, are now accepted as comprising a sizable group with a generally excellent prognosis, together with other quite specific features in their natural history. Because they are discussed in detail in another chapter in this volume, I will not have much to say about them here, except for two general comments. First, much of the discussion that follows concerning the relative prognostic importance of histologic type and grade pales in significance next to the distinction between borderline tumors and the corresponding invasive adenocarcinomas. Second, although the borderline tumors as a group are now fairly well understood, there are still several questions remaining regarding their classification and significance. These include the question of whether invasive carcinoma can be diagnosed without finding stromal invasion in the mucinous type, the criteria for diagnosis and clinical significance of variants other than serous and mucinous, the clinical significance (if any) of grading within the group of borderline tumors, and the significance of the histologic appearance of extraovarian "implants" associated with ovarian borderline tumors. These and other questions are currently the subject of active investigation, but the current literature still yields more questions than answers.

3 Clinicopathologic Staging of Ovarian Carcinoma

Virtually every article that has ever been published on ovarian cancer emphasizes the primacy of staging in the establishment of both a therapeutic regimen and the ultimate prognosis. The staging system of the International Federation of Gynaecology and Obstetrics (FIGO) is presented in Table 2.

---

[1] As exemplified in the Chapter by Professor Fox appearing in this volume.

Table 2. FIGO staging of carcinomas of the ovary

Stage I.   Growth limited to the ovaries
       Ia)   Growth limited to one ovary; no ascites;
       Ib)   Growth limited to both ovaries; no ascites;
       Ic)   Growth limited to one or both ovaries; ascites present or malignant cells in peritoneal washings.

Stage II.   Growth involving one or both ovaries with pelvic extension;
       IIa)   Extension and/or metastasis to the uterus and/or tubes only;
       IIb)   Extension to other pelvic tissues
       IIc)   Stage IIa or IIb plus ascites or positive peritoneal washings.

Stage III.   Growth involving one or both ovaries with intraperitoneal metastasis to the abdomen (including omentum, small intestine and its mesentery) and/or positive retroperitoneal nodes.

Stage IV.   Growth involving one or both ovaries with distant metastasis outside the peritoneal cavity.

Note: Stages Ia and Ib are subclassified (i) or (ii) depending upon the absence (i) or presence (ii) of tumor on the ovarian surface and/or capsular rupture

Unlike most other tumors, ovarian neoplasms are staged after surgery. Thus, the pathologist plays a decisive role in the staging process. Although the concept of the gynecologist and pathologist operating as a team in the management of ovarian cancer is discussed elsewhere in this volume, we must at least briefly mention here that the correct interpretation by the pathologist of histopathologic and cytological material obtained from outside the ovaries during a staging laparotomy will essentially determine the initial stage of an ovarian cancer, which in turn will in large measure influence the selection of the proper therapeutic regimen and the ultimate outcome.

It is thus important to remember that a number of benign lesions exist which enter into the differential diagnosis of metastatic ovarian cancer. These have been reviewed recently at the histologic level by FARHI and SILVERBERG (1982) and by COFFIN et al. (1985), and at the cytologic level by SNEIGE et al. (1986) and by SIDAWY and SILVERBERG (1987). Although a number of benign proliferative lesions can be confused with metastatic ovarian carcinoma, by far the most common of these is the condition known as *endosalpingiosis*, which is usually used today to define any proliferation of Mullerian-type epithelium on a peritoneal surface. As the name implies, these proliferations most often are of tubal epithelial type, and thus are most likely to be confused with metastases from carcinomas of serous type. Similar proliferations are also encountered in the capsule as well as the parenchyma of pelvic and paraontic lymph nodes, where they may also be confused by the unwary with metastatic ovarian cancer.

Endosalpingiosis is seen most commonly as small gray-white to yellow, firm, occasionally calcified nodules measuring no more than 2 mm in diameter each, within the omentum and cul-de-sac and on the serosal surfaces of the uterine corpus, ovaries, fallopian tubes, bowel, bladder and diaphragm. The microscopic appearance varies from small glands and cysts lined by a single layer of uniform cuboidal cells to complex papillary tufts with pseudostratification and tubal, endometrial, mucinous or even urothelial metaplasia. Calcification – often in the form of psammoma bodies – is common, as are chronic inflammation and fibrosis accompanying and entrapping the proliferating glandular elements. These stromal reactions may produce the false appearance of invasion, and so it is important to note the generally benign cytologic features of the cells lining the glands, cysts and papillae. In cytologic material as well – particularly in pelvic washings taken at the time of exploratory laparotomy – papillary proliferations and psammoma bodies may suggest the diagnosis of metastatic carcinoma, but the nuclear features in endosalpingiosis are benign.

Although ZINSSER and WHEELER (1982) suggested that the presence or absence of ovarian cancer was an important feature in the differential diagnosis between endosalpingiosis and metastatic carcinoma, McCAUGHEY et al. (1984) identified endosalpingiosis in 40% of their cases of borderline serous tumor of the ovary, and we have encountered it frequently in association with invasive ovarian carcinoma as well.

Another staging problem in which the role of the pathologist is important relates to the decision whether foci of cancer seen outside the ovaries represent metastatic disease or separate primary carcinomas. In the case of serous carcinoma, we know that multiple extraovarian primary cancers can occur, since they may be seen when the ovaries are uninvolved (TOBACMAN et al. 1982) or only minimally involved by microscopic foci of tumor arising from surface mesothelium (AUGUST et al. 1985). When an ovarian tumor mass is present, however, it makes little difference how the numerous peritoneal implants developed, since the prognosis and treatment are the same in any event.

With non-serous ovarian cancers, on the other hand, a single focus of extraovarian cancer of the same histologic type may be present elsewhere, and in this case the decision between a double primary and a solitary metastasis can be an important one. Probably the best known and most common situation of this sort involves the coexistence of endometrioid carcinoma of the ovary and primary carcinoma of the endometrium (EIFEL et al. 1982), but histologically similar mucinous carcinomas may be seen simultaneously involving ovary and endocervix or ovary and bowel, and transitional cell carcinomas are occasionally seen in both the ovary and the urinary tract. In each of these situations, the identification of a premalignant lesion or in situ carcinoma in the extraovarian location is the best evidence favoring separate primary origins. In endometrioid carcinoma involving both ovary and endometrium, it can also be assumed that both lesions are primary if the patient is young, both tumors are of low histologic grade, and invasion into the myometrium by the endometrial carcinoma is not seen (EIFEL et al. 1982).

4 Clinical Significance of Histologic Type

Even before the onset of deliberations by the committee that produced the WHO classification, it had been assumed for many years that the histologic type of invasive epithelial carcinoma bore a relationship to the prognosis for survival (DAY et al. 1975). In virtually every series ever published, undifferentiated carcinoma has had the poorest prognosis, and in most series this has been followed closely by serous carcinoma, with the other histologic types being relatively more favorable. Only in recent years, however, have more sophisticated analyses been published that simultaneously compared stage, grade, and other features. In addition, as new therapeutic modalities for ovarian carcinoma have developed rapidly within the past several years, it is of relatively little use to analyse the results of series in which these modalities were not utilized. Thus, the literature review to be undertaken here will emphasize those articles that have been published within the last five years.

As a preamble, however, we must first mention three articles published in 1975 which seemed to stimulate much of the interest in comparing the independent effect of histologic types and grades in ovarian carcinoma in subsequent years. DECKER et al. (1975) and DAY et al. (1975) both presented their data at a National Cancer Institute symposium, and both emphasized the prognostic importance of histologic grading as opposed to typing. Decker and his group reported on a series of 730 cases of epithelial carcinoma of the ovary treated at the Mayo Clinic between 1950 and 1965 (and therefore mostly prior to the development of modern chemotherapeutic regimens). Most of the tumors were classified as either serous (68%) or mucinous (21%), while only 5% were endometrioid and 6% "solid." Survival analyses compared only serous and mucinous carcinomas, since these were the most common types, and found that "stage for stage and grade for grade, the survival rate was not different." The grading system used was said to be a modification of the BRODERS (1926) system, and thus would be classified as cytologic rather than architectural. In this series, grading influenced survival both in early and late stages, and both for mucinous tumors alone and serous tumors alone.

In the same symposium, DAY et al. (1975) presented data on 250 cases of epithelial carcinoma that were reviewed by a single pathologist. Neither the dates nor the modalities of treatment were quoted, but it can be assumed that modern chemotherapy was not included to any major extent. The great majority (215 of 250) of all tumors were categorized as serous, leaving too few examples of other tumor types for adequate comparison, but mucinous carcinomas were noted to have a more favorable prognosis than the serous group. Again, both stage and grade were more important than type in this analysis.

SCULLY (1975b), in the subsequent discussion, pointed out one defect common to these two presentations, as well as to others subsequently published from these institutions (the Mayo Clinic and the M.D. Anderson Hospital and Tumor Institute), as well as from several other institutions. Neither presentation referred to "borderline tumors" or "carcinomas of low malignant potential", since these lesions were not separated as distinct entities in either of the institutions represented. Scully commented that he thought "from listening to the speakers and looking at some of the illustrations, what is considered borderline malignancy in the WHO classification is considered grade 1 or perhaps grade 2 carcinoma among the serous and mucinous tumors" in the classification presented from the two institutions. Since in our own material mucinous borderline tumors are seen as frequently as mucinous carcinomas, and serous borderline tumors with half the frequency of invasive serous carcinomas (KATSUBE et al.

1982), the inclusion of large numbers of borderline lesions, with their well documented favorable prognosis, would certainly guarantee a favorable prognostic significance for the grade 1 carcinomas in these reports.

Also in 1975, BARBER et al., published a paper which has been widely quoted subsequently. They separately analyzed two different grading systems, as well as histologic type and other pathologic features, in an attempt to determine which would serve best as prognostic indicators in ovarian cancer treated by surgery with or without radiotherapy. One of the grading systems was the Ewing modification of Broders grades and the other was nuclear grading, so both would be classified today as cytologic rather than architectural. Although it is difficult to be sure, there probably were no borderline tumors included in this series. The authors found again that stage was the single most important prognostic indicator. Both grading systems seemed to have some clinical validity, but the differences were not significant within each stage for serous carcinomas (the only group large enough to analyze separately). Among the histologic types, mucinous carcinoma had the best prognosis, and clear cell and undifferentiated carcinomas the worst.

Although numerous other articles pertinent to this discussion were published in the ensuing years, we shall now turn to 1982 to continue the discussion of the prognostic significance of histologic type. One of the largest series yet published analyzed 2,412 cases of ovarian carcinoma treated at the Radiumhemmet in Stockholm during the period 1958 to 1973 (BJÖRKHOLM et al. 1982). Treatment included single-agent chemotherapy in the more recent cases, but modern chemotherapeutic techniques were not employed. Borderline tumors were analyzed separately, and among the invasive carcinomas the most common types were serous (53%) and endometrioid (13%). In this series, mucinous and endometrioid carcinomas had a more favorable prognosis than clear cell and serous carcinomas, which in turn were more favorable than the anaplastic and "not otherwise specified" tumors. Multivariate analysis still revealed that histologic type was of prognostic significance, but grading was not considered as a factor in this series (except for separation of the borderline tumors, which uniformly showed superior survival statistics). Even among Stage Ia tumors only, the clear cell, serous and anaplastic carcinomas continued to have a less favorable prognosis.

Another series from Sweden published in the same year (SORBE et al. 1982) also confirmed the prognostic importance of histologic type, with mucinous, endometrioid, and "mesonephroid" (clear cell) carcinomas being more favorable than serous carcinomas, which in turn were more favorable than anaplastic carcinomas. Borderline tumors were analyzed separately, but appeared to be rather infrequent in this material. Probably only a small proportion of the patients were treated with modern chemotherapy. In this series, it was noted that most mucinous tumors were of low grade and low stage, while most serous carcinomas were of high grade and high stage. It was concluded that "grading is perhaps as important as tumor staging and is obviously superior to histologic type as a prognostic factor."

Also in 1982, DEMBO and BUSH reviewed a series of 430 patients with ovarian carcinoma, whose tumors were subtyped and graded by a single pathologist.

Borderline tumors were excluded, and treatment was nonuniform. The results were used to classify the carcinomas into a favorable group consisting of mucinous, endometrioid, clear cell, and well differentiated serous carcinomas, and an unfavorable group consisting of poorly differentiated serous and undifferentiated carcinomas. Multivariate analysis revealed a complex relationship between histologic type and grade, with the grade only being of prognostic significance within the category of serous carcinomas. However, the exact grading procedure utilized was not specified.

In 1983, SCHRAY et al. published their experience in 152 patients with stages I, II and III epithelial carcinoma who received radiation therapy as the sole postoperative treatment. Eighty-two percent of the cases were reviewed by a single pathologist. In this analysis, endometrioid carcinomas were more favorable than serous carcinomas, which in turn were more favorable than undifferentiated carcinomas at a statistically significant level. However, with multivariate analysis, tumor grade was the single most important feature and histologic type the least important.

Also in 1983, SIGURDSSON et al. reported another series of cases from Sweden, in which postoperative treatment consisted of no treatment, radiotherapy, single agent chemotherapy, or combined radiotherapy plus single-agent chemotherapy, depending upon the stage of the tumor and the presence or absence of capsular invasion or rupture. No borderline tumors were included in the study. The survival statistics were best for mucinous carcinomas and worst for anaplastic and unclassified carcinomas, with endometrioid, "mesonephroid," and serous carcinomas in an intermediate position. It was noted that 65% of the mucinous carcinomas were in early stage while 65% of the serous carcinomas were in advanced stage. Similarly, 78% of the mucinous carcinomas were well differentiated, versus only 40% of the endometrioid, 32% of the serous, and 13% of the "mesonephroid" tumors. Cox regression analysis revealed that grade was more significant than type in all cases except Stage III with bulky residual disease and Stage IV.

In 1984, GUTHRIE et al. reported a study of 656 patients with "early" ovarian cancer (defined as any tumor that had been totally excised at initial operation, and by analysis consisting more than 80% of stage I cases). Postoperative treatment, when given, consisted mostly of single agent chemotherapy. It was noted that clear cell carcinomas fared significantly worse regardless of stage. Mucinous carcinomas had a more favorable prognosis, but 73% of them were in Stage Ia. Carcinomas of borderline malignancy were analyzed separately, and no recurrences or deaths were seen among this group of 135 patients. As one might expect with "early" cancer, there were almost equal numbers of serous, mucinous and endometrioid carcinomas, and very few tumors with anaplastic or indeterminate histology. Also in 1984, MALKASIAN et al. updated the Mayo Clinic results with a report of 1938 cases of epithelial ovarian cancer treated between 1950 and 1979. Few cases were treated with modern chemotherapy, and as in other reports from this institution, borderline tumors were not considered separately. It was noted that mucinous carcinomas and carcinomas of mixed mucinous and serous type tended to be correlated with Grade I and Stage I and to have the most favorable prognosis, while serous and "not otherwise specified" carcinomas were least favorable. As in the 1975 analysis by DECKER et al. from this institution, it was noted that "for most histologic cell types, observed differences in survival were more apparent than real since the behavior of different cell types was similar when compared stage for stage and grade for grade."

NEIJT et al. (1984) reported a series of 186 patients with advanced epithelial ovarian carcinoma who were treated with one of two combination chemotherapy regimens. In this series (the first covered thus far in this review in which all patients received modern chemotherapy), histologic type was not significant either in predicting survival or in predicting response to chemotherapy.

In 1985, GERSHENSON et al. reported a series of 246 patients with advanced (Stages III and IV) epithelial ovarian cancer who underwent second-look laparotomy at the M.D. Anderson Hospital and Tumor Institute. Eighty-five of these patients had a negative second-look laparotomy, and were the subject of the published report. Sixty-five percent of the initial tumors in this group were of serous type. It was stated that cases of mixed histologic type did significantly worse, but no other differences were noted among the different histologic types. There had been no uniformity of treatment before second-look procedure.

In another report published in the same year (SWENERTON et al. 1985), a multivariate analysis of prognostic factors was performed on a series of 556 women with invasive epithelial carcinoma treated predominantly with radiotherapy and/or single alkylating agent chemotherapy following surgery. All cases were reviewed by a single pathologist, and borderline tumors were excluded. The most common tumour types included in the series were serous (380 cases) and mucinous (106 cases); few examples of other types were included. By univariate analysis there was a significant prognostic difference based on histologic type, with "mesonephric," endometrioid and mucinous carcinomas more favorable than serous carcinomas, and undifferentiated carcinoma having the worst prognosis. However, by multivariate analysis, histologic type was no longer of any prognostic significance.

Another report from the Radiumhemmet in Stockholm (EINHORN et al. 1985) analyzed multiple prognostic factors in 770 cases of invasive ovarian carcinoma treated during the period 1974 to 1979. Treatment was nonuniform, with various combinations of surgery, radiotherapy and chemotherapy being utilized. As in the previous report summarized above from the same institution (BJÖRKHOLM et al. 1982), endometrioid and mucinous carcinomas were associated with better survival than serous and "mesonephric" carcinomas, with anaplastic tumors the worst of all. In the present series, however, it was noted that only 16% of the serous carcinomas were in early stages at the time of initial diagnosis and treatment, as opposed to 39% of the mesonephric, 52% of the endometrioid, and 53% of the mucinous carcinomas. When the different histologic types were analyzed stage for stage, histology made no difference in survival in Stages IIB through IV, and an analysis of survival by histologic type in early stage lesions was not provided.

In one of the few articles to report a more favorable prognosis for serous than non-serous carcinomas, EDMONSON et al. (1985) reported on 187 women with Stage III and IV ovarian carcinoma who were treated with two multiagent chemotherapeutic regimens containing cisplatin. Although the tumors classified as serous did indeed have a significantly more favorable survival than all others, closer analysis reveals that almost half of the "others" were classified as undifferentiated carcinoma, with relatively small numbers of mucinous, endometrioid and clear cell carcinomas. Since these histologic types were not analyzed separately, we can make little of the data. It is also notable that this report comes from the Mayo Clinic, and thus the serous group (as well as the much smaller mucinous group) may contain a significant proportion of borderline tumors.

In another trial comparing two chemotherapeutic regimens containing cisplatin (CONTE et al. 1986), the familiar pattern of mucinous and endometrioid carcinomas faring more favorably than serous carcinomas, with undifferentiated carcinomas having the poorest prognosis, emerged again. There is no information presented to relate the histologic type to clinical stage in this report, but all cases were at least Stage Ic, and the great majority were in Stages III and IV, suggesting that the statistically significant differences in survival between histologic types may be real.

Three recent articles have reported on the relationship between histopathologic findings and other variables and the tumor status at second-look laparotomy following apparent complete clinical response after chemotherapy in epithelial ovarian carcinoma. PODRATZ et al. (1985), in a series of 135 patients treated at the Mayo Clinic, found that the original cell type of carcinoma did not significantly influence the findings at reexploration. However, SMIRZ et al. (1985), in a series of 88 patients, found that endometrioid carcinomas were less likely to have residual tumor found at second look than were serous and "not otherwise specified" carcinomas, with too few mucinous or clear cell carcinomas to be analyzed. Finally, MILLER et al. (1986), in another series of 88 patients, found with multivariate regression analysis that only initial and postsurgical maximal tumor diameter and histologic type were independently significant in predicting disease-free status. The unfavorable histologic type here was serous carcinoma, which comprised 62% of all cases, with the next most frequent subtype being adenocarcinoma not otherwise specified (22%).

In brief summary, the histologic type of invasive carcinoma was important in predicting survival and/or recurrence-free status in the great majority of the articles reviewed. With some exceptions, the usual pattern was for a favorable prognosis with mucinous and endometrioid carcinomas, a relatively unfavorable prognosis for serous carcinomas, and an extremely unfavorable prognosis for anaplastic or undifferentiated carcinomas. Clear cell or "mesonephric" carcinomas are grouped with the favorable tumors in about half of the reports and with the unfavorable ones in the other half, suggesting that their prognostic significance is intermediate or that they are so uncommon that few series comprise enough cases to arrive at a reasonable conclusion. "Adenocarcinoma not otherwise specified" usually falls into the less favorable category, confirming our own impression that this term is generally used for poorly differentiated carcinomas that are not totally anaplastic.

Although histologic type thus does seem to be of prognostic importance when considered alone, those studies in which multivariate statistical analysis was performed were almost uniform in finding it to be of less importance than other features, and in many instances of no importance at all (SCHRAY et al. 1983; SIGURDSSON et al. 1983; MALKASIAN et al. 1984; EINHORN et al. 1985; SWENERTON et al. 1985; MILLER et al. 1986). It thus behooves us to search for other pathologic features of possible prognostic significance, as well as to inquire into whether the histologic type of epithelial ovarian carcinoma does have some clinical significance other than in the assessment of prognosis.

5 Tumor Grade

One histologic feature which is believed by many authors to be a superior alternative to histologic type as a prognostic indicator is tumor grade. As mentioned above, the recent interest in tumor grade as a prognostic feature was stimulated initially by the independent contributions in 1975 of DECKER et al. and DAY et al. Both of these reports were enthusiastic about the use of histologic grading as a prognostic indicator, and presented data showing distinct differences in survival related to tumor grade, both overall and within specific stages and specific histologic types. DECKER et al. (1975) made it clear that the grading system they were using was a modification of the BRODERS (1926) system, in which Grade I corresponded to 0–25% of "undifferentiated cells" (whatever these are in adenocarcinomas), Grade 2 to 25–50%, Grade 3 to 50–75%, and Grade 4 to 75–100%. The report of DAY et al. did not specify the grading system used, other than to state that Grade I was equivalent to well differentiated, Grade II to moderately differentiated, and Grade III to poorly differentiated. SCULLY (1975b), in his discussion of these two presentations, mentioned as a common weakness of both the fact that tumors of borderline malignancy or low malignant potential were not eliminated from these series, and thus many of the "Grade I" and some "Grade II" tumors reported probably belonged in this category, which is well established to have an extremely favorable prognosis.

Some of the defects of these early studies were eliminated in the work of OZOLS et al. (1979, 1980), who separately analyzed two different grading systems in a small series of 82 cases of Stage III–IV epithelial ovarian cancer treated by chemotherapy (mostly multiagent but not including cisplatin). In the 1980 publication, the two grading systems were not only defined but also illustrated in a series of photomicrographs. One of four cytologic grades was assigned to each tumor based on a modification of the Broders system, and one of three pattern (architectural) grades was assigned based on the degree to which the tumor produced papillary or glandular structures versus solid cellular sheets. In addition, it was noted that 6 of the 82 patients had tumors of borderline malignancy.

In this study, a definite association was noted between the two grading systems, in that as the histologic pattern became more undifferentiated, the cytologic grade also increased. The authors commented that the poorly differentiated pattern grade included only cytologic Grades III and IV. The pattern grading system clearly divided the patients into two survival groups, with the 16 patients with well differentiated tumors (which included the 6 with borderline malignancy) demonstrating significantly better survival than the combined group of 49 patients with moderately and poorly differentiated tumors (the total is less than 82 patients because not all patients had enough tumor reviewed to assign a pattern grade). With the cytologic grading system, the authors reported that "it identified four groups with different survival outcomes", but in another portion of the manuscript they noted that "survival of patients with cytologic Grade III and IV lesions was essentially the same," and also admitted that cytologic Grade I comprised only four cases, all of which were borderline tumors. Thus, although this is the single manuscript that has probably had the most influence in the area of grading of ovarian carcinomas, it appears that the conclusion of the authors that cytologic grading is superior to pattern grading is very shaky when reviewed with a critical eye. A separate conclusion of the authors that will also merit further consideration was that "in contrast to survival, where patients with Grade IV tumors had the worst prognosis, this same group had a high overall response rate which was independent of either single-agent or combination chemotherapy."

In the same five-year period covered by the review above of the relation of histologic type of ovarian carcinoma to prognosis, even more reports explored the relationship between histologic grade and survival in this disease. Let us first examine once more the reports quoted above, to the extent that they commented on the significance of tumor grade as well as of tumor type. As mentioned above, DEMBO and BUSH (1982) stated that grade was a prognostically significant factor only in the subtype of serous carcinoma, whereas all mucinous, endometrioid and clear cell carcinomas were classified as favorable. They divided the serous carcinomas only into a well differentiated prognostically favorable and a poorly differentiated prognostically unfavorable group, and did not specify what grading procedure was used. Few if any of the patients in this series (treated between 1971 and 1976) received modern chemotherapy.

SORBE et al. (1982), however, stated that grade was the single most important prognostic factor in their series, with the differences in survival based on grade being significant in Stages I and II, and showing similar trends in Stages III and IV. The grade-based survival differences persisted with separate analyses of serous and mucinous carcinomas. Borderline tumors were excluded from this series, but treatment was not uniform, and cisplatin-based regimens do not appear to have been used. The grading system used was cytologic, and was defined in some detail but not illustrated; interestingly, grades were assigned from the least differentiated part of each tumor. Grade was clearly thought to be more important than histologic type by these authors.

SCHRAY et al. (1983) also concluded that grade was a more important prognostic feature than histologic type, and indeed was even more important than stage in their material. Grading was said to have "combined the architectural pattern and cytologic features," but was not otherwise defined. The patients in this series were treated with surgery and radiotherapy alone as initial treatment.

SIGURDSSON et al. (1983) also found that, with Cox regression analysis, tumor grade was almost always more significant as a prognostic factor than was histologic type. The only exceptions were in Stage III tumors with bulky residual disease and Stage IV. The exact grading system applied was again not specified, and the significant results were that well differentiated and moderately differentiated tumors combined did better than poorly differentiated ones. Postoperative treatment in this series included radiotherapy and/or single agent chemotherapy.

In the study of 656 patients with "early" ovarian cancer already quoted above, GUTHRIE et al. (1984), using an unspecified grading system, found that survival in well differentiated tumors was better than that in all others, but not at a statistically significant level. We do not know if borderline tumors were excluded, and most patients were treated with single-agent chemotherapy, not including cisplatin. Histologic type was also not particularly important in this series, with only clear cell carcinoma being said to have a significantly poorer prognosis.

MALKASIAN et al. (1984) confirmed previous studies from the Mayo Clinic in stating that tumor grade (determined cytologically) was more important than tumor type in assaying the prognosis of epithelial malignant tumors. Few patients in this series were treated with modern chemotherapy, and, as in other studies from this institution, the proportion of borderline tumors included among the Grade I carcinomas cannot be determined.

This latter criticism can also be applied to several other reports from the Mayo Clinic (PODRATZ et al. 1985; EDMONSON et al. 1985) and M.D. Anderson (GERSHENSON et al. 1985). The reports of PODRATZ et al. and GERSHENSON et al. both involved patients subjected to second-look laparotomy, and both found a relationship between pretreatment tumor grade and long-term survival. The grading system in the Podratz manuscript was cytologic, while in the Gershenson article grading was done by pattern. Treatment was nonuniform in both of these series although a significant proportion of patients in each did receive cisplatin-based chemotherapy. In the EDMONSON (1985) report from the Mayo Clinic, all patients did receive cisplatin-based chemotherapy, and all cases were in Stage III or IV. Moderately differentiated and poorly differentiated tumors showed almost identical survival statistics, while the relatively small proportion (about 10%) of well differentiated tumors did significantly better – but again we do not know how many of these were actually of borderline malignancy.

In another report of cisplatin-treated patients with advanced ovarian carcinoma (NEIJT et al. 1984), tumor grade (by cytologic criteria) was less important than stage and size of residual tumor after initial operation in predicting survival, but was important in predicting a response to chemotherapy, with 94% of the Grade IV tumors showing some response. Histologic type in this series did not predict either response or eventual survival.

In the study of SMIRZ et al. (1985), a somewhat different approach to grading was used, in that the criteria were predominantly architectural, but upgrading was done for a higher nuclear grade. This study was concerned with results at second-look laparotomy after various types of chemotherapy (about 60%

including cisplatin). In this series, there was no correlation of grade with either the presence or absence of residual disease at second-look or the eventual survival, although "grade O" (borderline) tumors were associated with superior survival.

Swenerton et al. (1985) excluded borderline tumors from their series, and graded by combined architectural and cytologic criteria, with the four grades used well characterized in the text. Treatment included surgery, radiotherapy, and single agent chemotherapy only. By univariate analysis both grade and histologic type were significant, but by multivariate analysis grade was prognostically significant in Stages I and II only, and histologic type was not significant in any stage. Einhorn et al. (1985) also reported that tumor differentiation (grading system not specified) was significant in early stage lesions only, with no prognostic significance in Stage III and no well differentiated tumors encountered in Stage IV. Since this report emanated from the Radiumhemmet, borderline tumors were probably excluded, although this is not stated in the manuscript. When analyzed by stage, tumor type seemed somewhat less important than tumor grade. Most patients in this series did not receive cisplatin.

Another series in which all patients did receive cisplatin was that of Conte et al. (1986). In this study, cytologic grading was used, and was found to have no prognostic significance. Histologic type was of importance in this series. The authors suggested that cisplatin treatment can overcome the prognostic significance of tumor grade reported in patients treated by other modalities.

Finally, among the reports previously reviewed, another group of patients initially treated predominantly with cisplatin and followed by second-look laparotomy was reported by Miller et al. (1986). Equal proportions of tumors (approximately 60%) were serous and poorly differentiated, although the grading procedure was not specified. Although the serous histology was significantly unfavorable by multivariate regression analysis, the tumor grade was not significant in determining the prognosis.

Several other reports in the last five years have commented on the prognostic significance of tumor grade but not of histologic type, and thus have not been discussed previously in the present report. Most of these series can be divided conveniently into those in which cisplatin was or was not used as first-line postoperative chemotherapy.

In the report of Klein et al. (1985), 110 patients with advanced ovarian carcinoma were treated with multiple chemotherapeutic regimens, but only 13 of these patients received cisplatin. The grading system applied was not specified, and tumor grade was not found to have a significant influence on survival. In the large series of Bruckner et al. (1985), advanced ovarian cancer was also treated with multiagent chemotherapy excluding cisplatin. The grading procedure used was again not specified. Well differentiated carcinomas were said to have a more favorable prognosis than moderately and poorly differentiated tumors combined, but the tumor grade was the least significant of all prognostic factors when Cox regression analysis was employed.

In two other reports in which Bruckner was also involved (Bruckner et al. 1983; Cohen et al. 1983), patients with advanced ovarian carcinoma were treated with cisplatin regimens. In the Cohen study, the grading system was not specified, but grade was not found to be important in influencing response as measured by second-look procedures. The authors concluded that cancer with aggressive features indicative of a short doubling time might be more vulnerable to effective chemotherapy than "indolent well-differentiated tumors," and that thus "the unfavorable influence of poor differentiation on outcome is a reflection of expectancy with no treatment or rather ineffective treatment." Indeed, in the report of BRUCKNER et al. (1983), there was actually longer survival noted in patients with poorly differentiated tumors (although again the grading system was not specified).

In a report which investigated specifically the effects of differentiation on prognosis in advanced ovarian carcinoma treated with cisplatin (JACOBS et al. 1982), an architectural grading system was employed, as well as separate breakdowns by cellular pleomorphism and mitotic activity. Although these three grading systems showed good interrelationships with each other, there was no relation between any of them and either survival or response to chemotherapy.

A few recent reports of large series include some but not all patients treated with cisplatin. In the series of WHARTON et al. (1984), 68 of the 395 patients with advanced ovarian were treated with cisplatin alone or in combination. A "pattern" (architectural) grading system was investigated, but Grade I probably induced carcinomas of low malignant potential. There was no separate analysis for histologic type. Grading was considered to be significant for longtime survival with all chemotherapeutic regimens, but the cisplatin-based regimens were not considered separately.

In the series of EDWARDS et al. (1983) – which like the proceding report, also emanated from M.D. Anderson – half of the 169 patients with advanced ovarian cancer were treated with a cisplatin-based regimen. A pattern grading system was used, and Grade I was found to be superior prognostically to Grades II and III combined. No mention was made of any differences based on grade between patients who were treated with or without cisplatin.

Another report in which some but not all patients were treated with cisplatin is that of CAIN et al. (1986). This series consisted of patients with no clinical residual disease following chemotherapy, who were subjected to second-look laparotomy. It was noted that the only correlations with the presence of residual disease at second look were the initial stage and the condition of residual tumor following initial surgery. Both histologic and cytologic grading were done, and neither correlated with the second-look findings, although survival after the second-look procedure in patients found to have residual disease did correlate with the cytologic grade of initial tumor.

Two other recent studies featured different approaches. CHEN and LEE (1984) reported a small series of patients with ovarian cancer in different stages who underwent retroperitoneal lymph node dissection. The tumors were graded according to the FIGO classification, and thus the grading was architectural. Grade III histology was found to be associated with the presence of lymph node metastases, as were the presence of lymphatic/vascular space invasion and the absence of notable lymphatic infiltration in the tumors.

The study of DEMOPOULUS et al. (1984) was unique in that it analyzed only patients with serous carcinomas. Postoperative treatment was variable, with some patients receiving cisplatin. Sixty-six percent of cases were in Stages III and IV, while 76% had Grade II and III tumors (graded by pattern). There was a good association between stage and grade. The tumor grade was found to be significant in its relation to survival "even after adjusting for stage", but the exact adjusted figures were not presented in the report.

In summary, despite the profusion of recent studies on the relationship of tumor grade to survival, most of these studies are difficult to interpret because of one or more confounding features, including: (1) the inclusion of borderline tumors in many of the series in which Grade I tumors are found to be prognostically favorable; (2) lack of specification of the exact grading system used and/or lack of grading by a single pathologist; and (3) absence of uniform treatment for all patients in a series. About the only conclusion that seems clear from the present review is that, in patients treated with cisplatin-based regimens, no system of tumor grading appears to be of major prognostic significance. In patients treated without cisplatin, grading *may* be of significance, but we suspect that if the borderline tumors are segregated out at one end of the spectrum, and undifferentiated carcinomas at the other end, grading of the differentiated invasive carcinomas that remain will probably have a fairly minor effect.

6 Reproducibility of Diagnostic and Grading Criteria

In most of the reports review above, the assumption was made tacitly that both the histologic subtyping and the architectural or cytologic grading of epithelial ovarian tumors were uniform among the pathologists in a single institution or, in some cases, multiple institutions. In fact, however, only a few studies have been designed to test that hypothesis.

HERNANDEZ et al. (1984) reported a study in which two pathologists independently reviewed a series of 68 malignant epithelial ovarian tumors. The interobserver agreement rate was 60% for histologic type and 66% for grade. The differences in typing of these tumors was noted to be due to tumor heterogeneity (more than one histologic type within a single tumor) and the differential diagnosis beween serous and undifferentiated carcinomas. With respect to grade, about 20% of the disagreements concerned the differential diagnosis between invasive carcinoma and carcinoma of low malignant potential, while the others were attributed to the fact that one observer used architectural criteria and the other utilized mitotic counts in arriving at the final grade.

The other recent work in this field has been published by BAAK and his colleagues (1982, 1986a, 1986b). In the first of these studies, 49 mucinous ovarian tumors were reviewed by four pathologists. There was disagreement in 25% of the cases, predominantly concerning the distinction between tumors of low malignant potential and invasive carcinomas (nine cases) or between tumors of low malignant potential and benign cystadenomas (two cases). In a subsequent larger study (BAAK et al. 1986b), 198 cases were evaluated independently by four different gynecologic pathologists. Histologic typing was done using the WHO classification, and the tumors were graded as benign, borderline or malignant (well, moderately or poorly differentiated). Since the slides were evaluated twice (at approximately a 1-year interval) by each pathologist, both interobserver and intraobserver reproducibility were evaluated. Histologic typing in general was less consistent than grading, but complete agreement was rare in either determination. Disagreements in histologic typing could generally be resolved after panel discussions, but it was pointed out that only a limited number of tumor types were utilized in the study. With histologic grading, complete agreement among all four pathologists was reached in only 18.7% of cases in the first round and 32.8% in the second. Intraobserver agreement in grading between the two rounds varied from 86% for the internally most consistent pathologist to 62% for the pathologist with the least reproducibility. Since only one slide per case was used, it was noted that the results might have been even worse had a complete set of slides from each tumor been utilized. The authors pointed out in their discussion that "the grading and typing of ovarian tumors is not a end in itself: the aim is to provide prognostic information," and also stated that "further studies are required to determine whether grading differences truly reflect prognostic differences."

In a companion study, BAAK et al. (1986a) attempted to evaluate the decision-making criteria employed by the four study pathologists in the grading process. They noted that the sets of histologic and cytologic features with the greatest correlation with the tumor grades assigned differed among the pathologists, probably indicating that the observers used different features in their grading processes. There was never a complete correlation, however, between any of the microscopic features investigated and the eventual grades assigned by the different pathologists. Thus, either the relationships are nonlinear, the grading process is influenced by random subjective factors, or both.

These few studies indicate that the problems encountered in attempting to relate histologic type and grade to prognosis in ovarian tumors may be at least in part the result of interpathologist – or even intrapathologist – diagnostic disagreement. At the very least, we should demand that a single pathologist review all the cases in any study on this subject before we agree to take the results seriously. The reports of such studies should also state in detail the histopathologic criteria utilized, so that these can be evaluated and (if advisable) duplicated by other pathologists dealing with these tumors.

7 Nonhistologic Techniques

Because of the confusion discussed above concerning the prognostic significance of histologic evaluations of ovarian cancers, we should briefly consider the possibility that nonhistologic techniques may be of equal or greater value, although a complete discussion of these is beyond the scope of the present review. Determinations of ploidy have been shown to be related to survival in several different studies, regardless of whether the determination was made by Feulgen staining of paraffin-embedded tumor tissues (ERHARDT et al. 1984), flow cytometry of paraffin-embedded tumor tissues (FRIEDLANDER et al. 1984), or flow cytometry of fresh tumor tissues (VOLM et al. 1985). The latter report also showed that studies of cell proliferation and short-term cell culture with specific chemotherapeutic agents were also useful in predicting both response to therapy and eventual survival. Other studies (IVERSON et al. 1986) have also demonstrated that tumor tissue analysis for estrogen and progesterone receptors can yield useful prognostic information. Studies of immunity, tumor markers, and gene probes also may all be of considerable value in the future.

8 Current Recommendations

Upon the receipt of an ovarian epithelial tumor in the laboratory, what then is the pathologist to do in terms of making his report clinically meaningful, considering the uncertainties that we have already discussed? First of all, it seems reasonable to expect a correct categorization of the tumor as benign, borderline or invasive carcinoma. It is also obviously important (as discussed above) to characterize correctly any mesothelial or epithelial proliferations – benign, borderline or invasive carcinoma – that may be submitted as products of a staging laparotomy. In many cases of disseminated disease, the sources of the tumor specimens may not be identifiable by either the gynecologist or the pathologist, but certainly every attempt should be made to prove the existence of an ovarian primary site if one exists, as well as to rule out the possibility that a tumor in the ovary may actually be metastatic from another site. When tumor is present in another viscus as well as one or both ovaries, an opinion should be expressed as to whether this situation represents a single primary with metastatic dissemination or multiple primary cancers without obvious dissemination, even if the best opinion is that it is impossible to resolve the issue.

Both the maximal diameter of the ovarian primary tumor or tumors and that of the largest extraovarian tumor mass resected should be reported. Particularly in early stage lesions, the condition of the ovarian capsule (ruptured, tumor on surface, or neither) should be stated, although the significance of this finding is still debated (DEMOPOULOS et al. 1984; EINHORN et al. 1985; SIGURDSSON et al. 1983). The prognostic significance of such factors as lymphatic or vascular space invasion, host lymphoid response, tumor fibrosis and necrosis is even less well characterized (BARBER et al. 1975; CHEN and LEE 1984), and thus comments related to these findings are probably of limited use unless they are part of a specific research protocol.

When we arrive at the ultimate questions of histologic typing and grading among the invasive carcinomas, it is clearly preferable to state both the type and grade in as clear and reproducible a manner as possible, since our literature review certainly indicates that we cannot definitely rule out the prognostic significance of either. Criteria for histologic typing are well defined in the WHO classification and standard textbooks, and require little amplification here. We should mention, however, that both mixed types and undifferentiated carcinomas should be diagnosed liberally, with the major and minor components always specified in the former situation. In the case of undifferentiated carcinoma, the pathologist should remember that a single mucin globule does not place an otherwise anaplastic tumor into the mucinous category, nor does a papilla or psammoma body change the diagnosis to serous carcinoma, since tumors with this scanty evidence of differentiation will clearly behave like other undifferentiated carcinomas.

We believe that histological typing of ovarian tumors will remain important even if its prognostic value is confirmed by future studies to be limited, since other useful information is also provided by the histologic type. For example, bilaterality rates vary considerably among the different histologic types, and this can be an important consideration in planning the approach to the contralateral ovary, particularly in a young woman with a borderline tumor. Ovarian epithelial tumors of different types also vary considerably in size, with the mucinous category invariably being the largest (KATSUBE et al. 1982). Finally, a correct assessment of the histologic type of epithelial cancer being considered should lead to an appropriate differential diagnosis – for example, consideration of an endometrial primary, and occasionally of a Sertoli cell tumor, in endometrioid carcinoma; the possibility of a bowel primary with mucinous carcinomas and a urothelial primary with ovarian transitional cell carcinomas; the differential diagnosis of endodermal sinus tumor when considering clear cell carcinoma, particularly in a young patient; and the possibility of an extraovarian primary site in serous carcinoma when the specimen submitted is not identifiable as ovary.

With regard to grading, the same statement made above about undifferentiated carcinoma should apply, since this tumor is clearly outside the spectrum of those differentiated carcinomas that should be graded. The same statement can be made for borderline or low malignant potential lesions, which should be clearly separated from low-grade invasive carcinomas. Within the spectrum of the differentiated invasive carcinomas, we recommend a separation into three grades, which may be designated Grades I, II and III, or well, moderately and poorly differentiated. We have chosen to illustrate in Fig. 1 and Fig. 2 our application of these grades both architecturally and cytologically to serous carcinomas, since these are in our experience (KATSUBE et al. 1982) and that of others the most common type of invasive epithelial cancer. Although we use architectural (pattern) grading in our own reports, we will upgrade a Grade I tumor to Grade II if the nuclei are uncharacteristically anaplastic.

In grading endometrioid carcinomas, we utilize the Gynecologic Oncology Group modification of the International Federation of Gynecology and Obstetrics (FIGO) grading system for carcinoma of the endometrium, in which Grade I tumors grow almost exclusively in a glandular and/or papillary pattern, with less than 5% solid sheets of cells; Grade II carcinomas display between 5 and 50% solid tumor growth; and Grade III tumors are more than half solid. Squamous elements – which by definition are solid – are considered outside this grading system.

We have less personal experience in grading the other types of epithelial cancers, since we encounter them much less frequently. However, a few general comments can be made here. First, we find that nearly all the mucinous carcino-

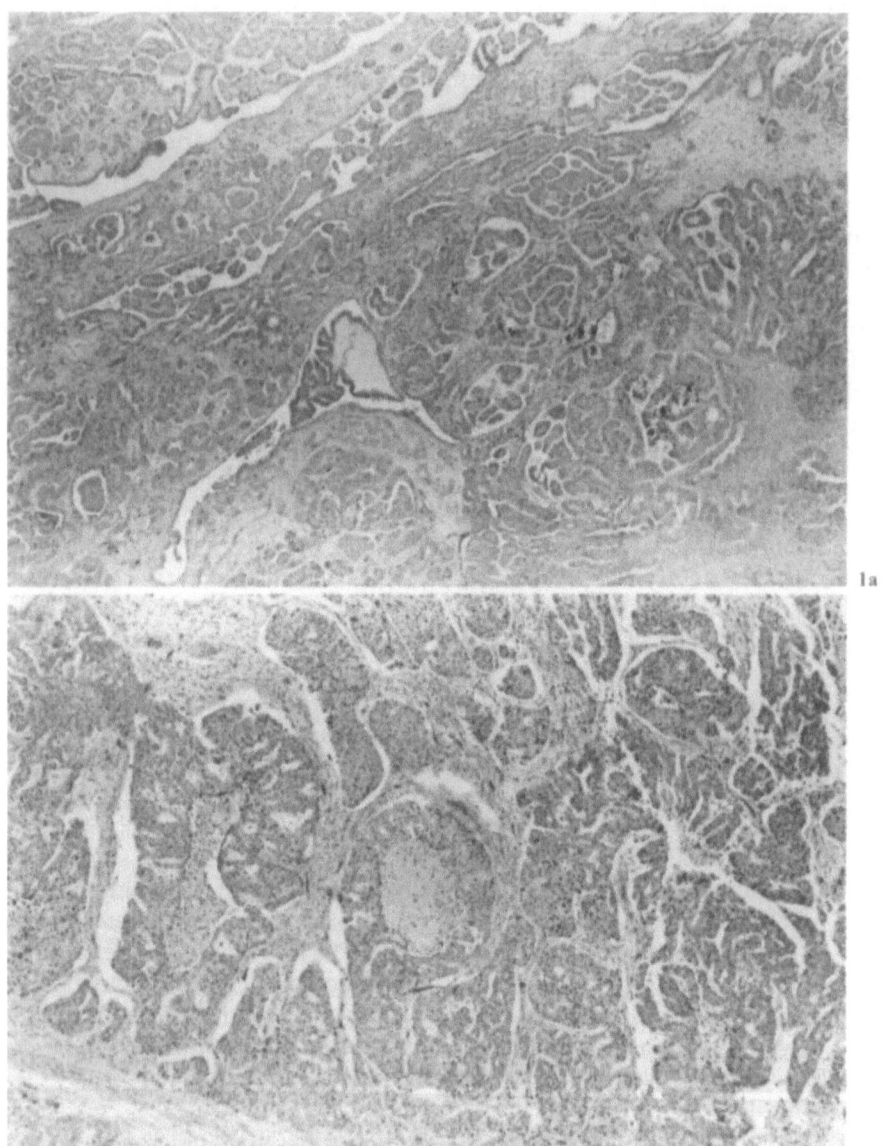

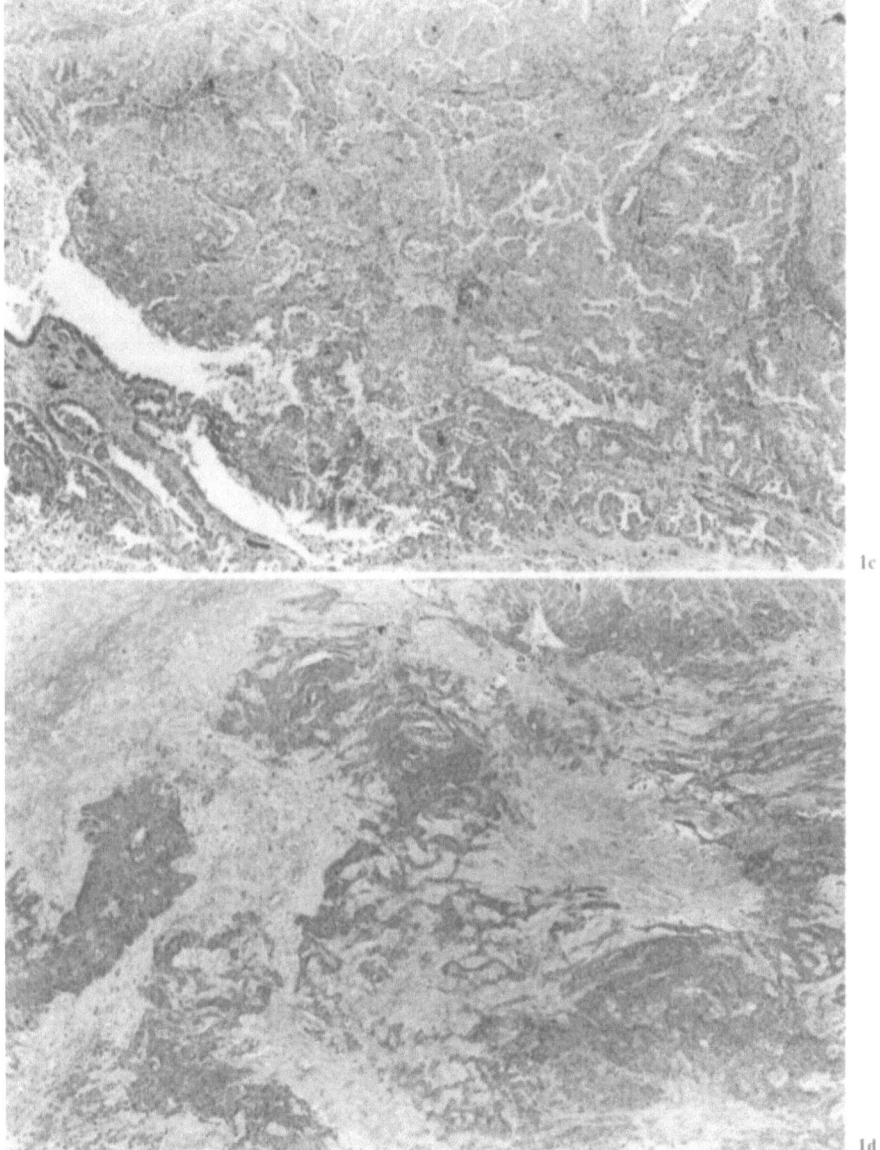

Fig. 1a–d. Architectural (pattern) grading of invasive serous carcinoma. **a** Grade I (well differentiated) tumor forms papillae with scattered psammoma bodies; no solid growth pattern is seen. **b** Grade II (moderately differentiated) carcinoma shows some solid tumor sheets, but is predominantly papilloglandular; the nonuniform and slit-like appearance of most of the lumina distinguish this from endometrioid carcinoma, which would have more uniform and rounded lumina. **c** Grade III (poorly differentiated) pattern is largely solid, but still includes slit-like lumina and some papillae. **d** A field of undifferentiated carcinoma, shown for comparison, is essentially entirely solid; since this field occurred in a tumor which elsewhere was predominantly serous, the overall diagnosis was still serous carcinoma. All magnifications are × 120

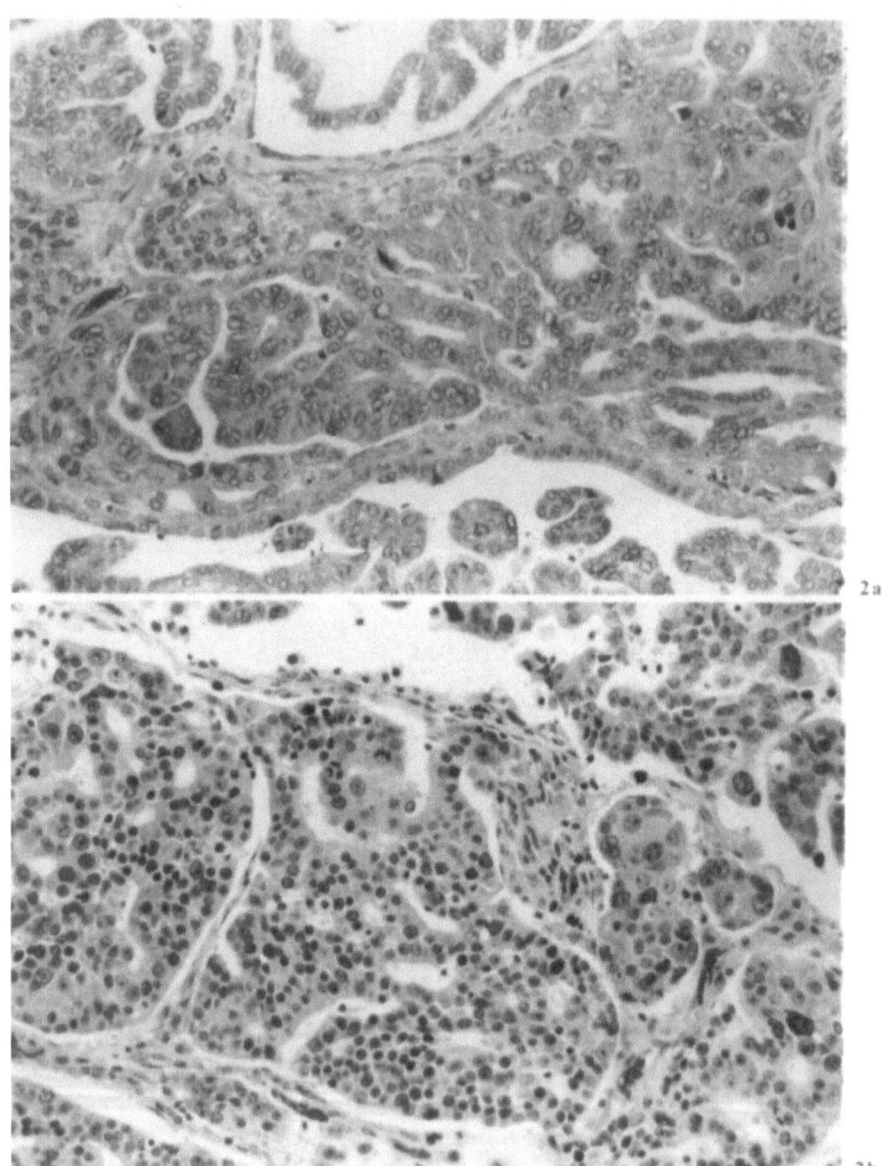

2 a

2 b

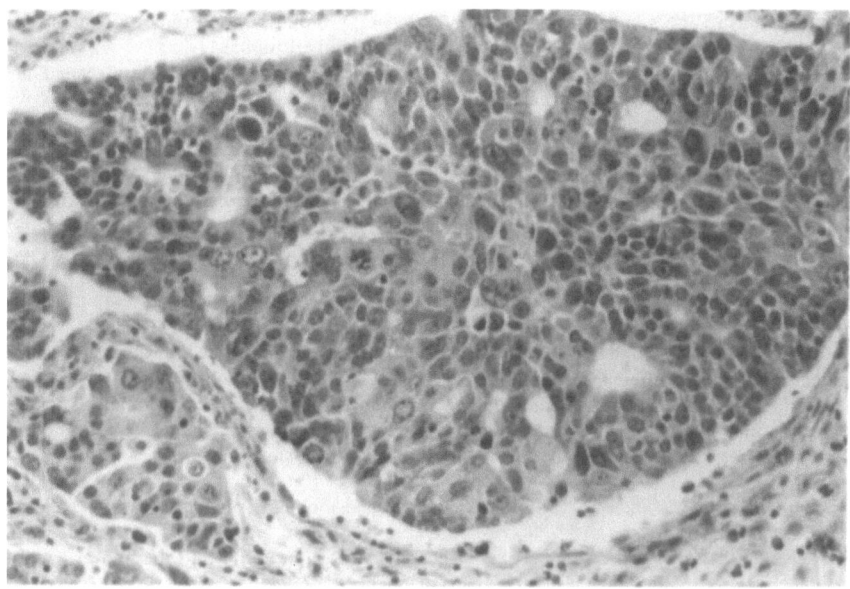

Fig. 2a–c. Cytological grading of invasive serous carcinoma. **a** Grade I (well differentiated) field shows uniform nuclei without prominent nucleoli, marked hyperchromatism, or numerous mitotic figures. **b** Grade II (moderately differentiated) focus with mostly small uniform nuclei; about 30% of nuclei are large, irregular and hyperchromatic; several mitotic figures are seen. **c** Grade III (poorly differentiated) field in which anisonucleosis, hyperchromatism and prominent nucleoli are the rule, giant and/or multiple nuclei are present in several cells, and an atypical mitosis is seen slightly left of center. All magnifications are × 480

mas that we encounter are moderately differentiated (Grade II), since our Grade I mucinous tumors are usually of low malignant potential and the Grade III ones often turn out to be metastatic from the gastro-intestinal tract. Clear cell carcinomas are almost aways poorly differentiated at the cytologic level and thus receive a final Grade of II or III when we upgrade our Grade I tumors for cytologic anaplasia as described above. We are far from convinced that the distinction between a Grade II and a Grade III clear cell carcinoma is of any clinical significance whatsoever. Finally, with respect to the rare carcinomas of urothelial type, we are impressed with the system of AUSTIN and NORRIS (1987), in which these lesions are designated as malignant Brenner tumors if benign or proliferating Brenner elements are found, and transitional cell carcinomas if the low-grade counterparts are absent, with the malignant Brenner tumors having by far the better prognosis of the two groups.

References

August CZ, Murad TM, Newton M (1985) Multiple focal extraovarian serous carcinoma. Int J Gynecol Pathol 4:11–23
Austin RM, Norris HJ (1987) Malignant Brenner tumor and transitional cell carcinoma of the ovary: A comparison. Int J Gynecol Pathol 6:29–39

Baak JPA, Delemarre JFM, Langley FA, Talerman A (1986a) Grading ovarian tumors: Evaluation of decision making by different pathologists. Anal Quant Cytol Histol 8:349–353

Baak JPA, Langley FA, Talerman A, Delamarre JFM (1986b) Interpathologist disagreement in ovarian tumor grading and typing. Anal Quant Cytol Histol 8:354–357

Baak JPA, Lindeman J, Overdiep SH, Langley FA (1982) Disagreement of histopathological diagnoses of different pathologists in ovarian tumours – with some theoretical considerations. Eur J Obstet Gynecol Reprod Biol 13:51–55

Barber HRK, Sommers SC, Snyder R, Kwon TH (1975) Histologic and nuclear grading and stromal reactions as indices for prognosis in ovarian cancer. Am J Obstet Gynecol 121:795–807

Björkholm E, Pettersson F, Einhorn N et al. (1982) Long-term follow-up and prognostic factors in ovarian carcinoma: The Radiumhemmet series 1958 to 1973. Acta Radiol Oncol 21 Fasc 6:413–419

Broders AC (1926) Carcinoma: Grading and practical application. Arch Pathol 2:376–380

Bruckner HW, Cohen CJ, Goldberg JD et al. (1983) Cisplatin regimens and improved prognosis of patients with poorly differentiated ovarian cancer. Am J Obstet Gynecol 145:653–658

Bruckner HW, Dinse GE, Davis TE et al. (1985) A randomized comparison of cyclophosphamide, Adriamycin, and 5-fluorouracil with triethylenethiophosphoramide and methotrexate, both as sequential and as fixed rotational treatment in patients with advanced ovarian cancer. Cancer 55:26–40

Cain JM, Saigo PE, Pierce VK, et al. (1986) A review of second-look laparotomy for ovarian cancer. Gynecol Oncol 23:14–25

Chen SS, Lee L (1984) Prognostic significance of morphology of tumor and retroperitoneal lymph nodes in epithelial carcinoma of the ovary. Gynecol Oncol 18:87–93

Coffin CM, Adcock LL, Dehner LP (1985) The second-look operation for ovarian neoplasms: A study of 85 cases emphasizing cytologic and histologic problems. Int J Gynecol Pathol 4:97–109

Cohen CJ, Goldberg JD, Holland JF et al. (1983) Improved therapy with cisplatin regimens for patients with ovarian carcinoma (FIGO Stages III and IV) as measured by surgical end-staging (second-look operation). Am J Obstet Gynecol 145:955–967

Conte PF, Bruzzone M, Chiara S et al. (1986) A randomized trial comparing cisplatin plus cyclophosphamide versus cisplatin, doxorubicin, and cyclophosphamide in advanced ovarian cancer. J Clin Oncol 4:965–971

Day TG Jr, Gallager HS, Rutledge FN (1975) Epithelial carcinoma of the ovary: Prognostic importance of histologic grade. Cancer Inst Monogr 42:15–18

Decker DG, Malkasian GD Jr, Taylor WF (1975) Prognostic importance of histologic grading in ovarian carcinoma. Nat Cancer Inst Monogr 42:9–11

Dembo AJ, Bush RS (1982) Current concepts in cancer: Ovary – Treatment for Stages III and IV: Choice of postoperative therapy based on prognostic factors. Int J Rad Oncol Biol Phys 8:893–897

Demopoulos RI, Bigelow B, Blaustein A et al. (1984) Characterization and survival of patients with serous cystadenocarcinoma of the ovaries. Obstet Gynecol 64:557–563

Edmonson JH, McCormack GW, Fleming TR et al. (1985) Comparison of cyclophosphamide plus cisplatin versus hexamethylmelamine, cyclophosphamide, doxorubicin, and cisplatin in combination as initial chemotherapy for Stage III and IV ovarian carcinomas. Cancer Treat Rep 69:1243–1248

Edwards CL, Herson J, Gershenson DM et al. (1983) A prospective randomized clinical trial of melphalan and cis-platinum versus hexamethylmelamine, Adriamycin, and cyclophosphamide in advanced ovarian cancer. Gynecol Oncol 15:261–277

Eifel P, Hendrickson M, Ross J et al. (1982) Simultaneous presentation of carcinoma involving the ovary and the uterine corpus. Cancer 50:163–170

Einhorn N, Nilsson BO, Sjovall K (1985) Factors influencing survival in carcinoma of the ovary. Study from a well-defined Swedish population. Cancer 55:2019–2025

Erhardt K, Auer G, Bjorkholm E et al. (1984) Prognostic significance of nuclear DNA content in serous ovarian tumors. Cancer Res 44:2198–2202

Farhi DC, Silverberg SG (1982) Pseudometastases in female genital cancer. Pathol Annu 17(1):47–76

Friedlander ML, Hedley DW, Taylor IW et al. (1984) Influence of cellular DNA content on survival in advanced ovarian cancer. Cancer Res 44:397–400

Gershenson DM, Copeland LJ, Wharton JT et al. (1985) Prognosis of surgically determined complete responders in advanced ovarian cancer. Cancer 55:1129–1135

Guthrie D, Davy MLJ, Philips PR (1984) A study of 656 patients with "early" ovarian cancer. Gynecol Oncol 17:363–369

Hernandez E, Bhagavan BS, Parmley TH, Rosenshein NB (1984) Interobserver variability in the interpretation of epithelial ovarian cancer. Gynecol Oncol 17:117–123

Iverson OE, Skaarland E, Utaaker E (1986) Steroid receptor content in human tumors: Survival of patients with ovarian carcinoma related to steroid receptor content. Gynecol Oncol 23:65–76

Jacobs AJ, Deligdish L, Deppe G, Cohen CJ (1982) Histologic correlates of virulence in ovarian adenocarcinoma. I. Effects of differentiation. Am J Obstet Gynecol 143:574–580

Katsube Y, Berg JW, Silverberg SG (1982) Epidemiologic pathology of ovarian tumors: A histopathologic review of primary ovarian neoplasms diagnosed in the Denver Standard Metropolitan Area, 1 July–31 December 1969 and 1 July–31 December 1979. Int J Gynecol Pathol 1:3–16

Klein B, Falkson G, Smit CF (1985) Advanced ovarian carcinoma: Factors influencing survival. Cancer 55:1829–1834

Malkasian GD Jr, Melton LJ III, O'Brien PC, Greene MH (1984) Prognostic significance of histologic classification and grading of epithelial malignancies of the ovary. Am J Obstet Gynecol 149:274–284

McCaughey WTE, Kirk ME, Lester W, Dardick I (1984) Peritoneal epithelial lesions associated with proliferative serous tumors of ovary. Histopathology 8:195–208

Miller DS, Ballon SC, Teng NNH et al. (1986) A critical reassessment of second-look laparotomy in epithelial ovarian carcinoma. Cancer 57:530–535

Neijt JP, ten Bokkel Huinink WW, van der Burgmel et al. (1984) Randomised trial comparing two combination chemotherapy regimens (Hexa-CAF vs CHAP-5) in advanced ovarian carcinoma. Lancet 2:594–600

Ozols RF, Garvin AJ, Costa J et al. (1979) Histologic grade in advance ovarian cancer. Cancer Treat Rep 63:255–263

Ozols RF, Garvin AJ, Costa J et al. (1980) Advanced ovarian cancer: Correlation of histologic grade with response to therapy and survival. Cancer 45:572–581

Podratz KC, Malkasian GD Jr, Hilton JF et al. (1985) Second-look laparotomy in ovarian cancer: Evaluation of pathologic variables. Am J Obstet Gynecol 152:230–238

Schray M, Martinez A, Cox R, Ballon S (1983) Radiotherapy in epithelial ovarian cancer: Analysis of prognostic factor based on long-term experience. Obstet Gynecol 62:373–382

Scully RE (1975a) World Health Organization Classification and Nomenclature of Ovarian Cancer. Nat Cancer Monogr 42:5–7

Scully RE (1975b) Discussion. Nat Cancer Inst Monogr 42:19–21

Serov SF, Scully RE, Sobin LH (1973) International Histological Classification of Tumours. No. 9, Histological Typing of Ovarian Tumours. Geneva, World Health Organization

Sidawy MS, Silverberg SG (1987) Endosalpingiosis in female peritoneal washings. A diagnostic pitfall. Int J Gynecol Pathol 6:340–346

Sigurdsson K, Alm P, Gullberg B (1983) Prognostic factors in malignant epithelial ovarian tumors. Gynecol Oncol 15:370–380

Smirz LR, Stehman FB, Ulbright TM et al. (1985) Second-look laporatomy after chemotherapy in the management of ovarian malignancy. Am J Obstet Gynecol 152:661–668

Sneige N, Fernandez T, Copeland LJ, Katz RL (1986) Müllerian inclusions in peritoneal washings: Potential source of error in cytologic diagnosis. Acta Cytol 30:271–276

Sorbe B, Frankendal BO, Veress B (1982) Importance of histologic grading in the prognosis of epithelial ovarian carcinoma. Obstet Gynecol 59:576–582

Swenerton KD, Hislop TG, Spinelli J et al. (1985) Ovarian carcinoma: A multivariate analysis of prognostic factors. Obstet Gynecol 65:264–270

Tobacman JK, Tucker MA, Kase R et al. (1982) Intra-abdominal carcinomatosis after prophylactic oophorectomy in ovarian – cancer – prone families. Lancet 2:795

Volm M, Brüggermann A, Günther M et al. (1985) Prognostic relevance of ploidy, proliferation, and resistance-predictive tests in ovarian carcinoma. Cancer Res 45:5180–5185

Wharton JT, Edwards CL, Rutledge FN (1984) Long-term survival after chemotherapy for advanced epithelial ovarian carcinoma. Am J Obstet Gynecol 148:997–1005

Zinsser KR, Wheeler JE (1982) Endosalpingiosis in the omentum. A study of autopsy and surgical material. Am J Surg Pathol 6:109–117

The Concept of Borderline Malignancy in Ovarian Tumours: A Reappraisal

H. Fox

1 Introduction

It is widely, though not universally, agreed that some epithelial ovarian tumours are neither fully benign nor overtly malignant, such neoplasms being put into a separate category of "ovarian epithelial tumours of borderline malignancy". Acceptance of this concept does, however, raise a number of questions:

i. What is the best terminology for these neoplasms?
ii. How should they be defined?
iii. Are serous tumours of borderline malignancy biologically equivalent to mucinous neoplasms of borderline malignancy and should the borderline category be extended to include some Brenner, endometrioid and clear cell tumours?
iv. Is there a continuous spectrum between benign and malignant ovarian epithelial tumours of which the borderline group is simply a segment or, alternatively, is this a discontinuous range with borderline tumours forming a discrete biological entity?
v. How should borderline tumours be treated?

It is the aim of this chapter to describe the pathology of ovarian epithelial tumours of borderline malignancy and to consider, though not necessarily to answer, the above questions.

2 Nomenclature

The term „tumour of borderline malignancy" is, despite its imperfections, the least objectionable of all the proposed forms of nomenclature for those neoplasms which lie in the grey hinterland between the orderly, controlled proliferation of benign neoplasia and the unrestrained cellular anarchy of true malignancy. It is true that the word „borderline" hints at uncertainty but it nevertheless accurately describes the somewhat ambivalent nature of these tumours: the term does not, however, indicate any indecision on the pathologist's part as to wether a particular tumour is benign or malignant. There is no justification for the claim that „there are no borderline tumours but only borderline pathologists" for the diagnosis of an ovarian tumour of borderline malignancy is a positive statement by the pathologist and does not represent an attempt to elevate pathological indecision into a nosological entity.

Many other names have, of course, been used to describe these neoplasms. The term "tumours of low grade malignancy" is often employed but has also frequently been used to describe well differentiated and slowly growing, but unequivocally malignant, neoplasms elsewhere in the body and carries with it the implication that borderline tumours are simply very well differentiated adenocarcinomas, thus denying their exclusive character. Some use the term "adenocarcinomas of low malignant potential" but this nomenclature suffers from the dual drawbacks of being biologically meaningless and of indicating that borderline tumours are a variant form of adenocarcinoma. The expression "tumours of low malignant potential" could equally well be applied to benign tumours which occasionally undergo malignant change whilst the term "proliferating epithelial tumour" retains its adherents despite the obvious fact that all neoplasms, whether benign or malignant, are formed by proliferating cells.

3 Definition

In the World Health Organization classification of ovarian neoplasms (SEROV et al. 1973) a borderline tumour is defined as "one which has some, but not all, of the morphological features of malignancy: those present include, in varying combinations, stratification of epithelial cells, apparent detachment of cellular clusters from their site of origin and mitotic figures and nuclear abnormalities intermediate between those of clearly benign and unquestionably malignant tumours of a similar cell type: on the other hand, obvious invasion of the stroma is lacking".

This description has all the characteristics, and drawbacks, of a definition drawn up by a committee and evades answering all the difficult questions.

It does not, for example, elaborate on the degree of nuclear abnormality and mitotic activity which can be classed as "intermediate" between benign and malignant tumours, does not indicate in precise terms what is meant by "obvious" stromal invasion and does not sufficiently stress that lack of stromal invasion is of prime diagnostic importance. This latter deficiency has, not unreasonably, been exploited by some who maintain that, particularly in the case of mucinous tumours, a non-invasive tumour can be classed as an adenocarcinoma if it shows marked epithelial abnormalities and cytological atypia (HART and NORRIS 1973; HART 1977). This approach is, to some extent, a reaction to the difficulties that may be encountered in deciding whether stromal invasion is present or not and in response to this difficulty there has been an increasing tendency to insist on a lack of "destructive" rather than "obvious" invasion. The term "destructive" has not been adequately defined in this context and it is well recognised that tumours in other sites, such as adenocarcinomas of the large bowel, may show invasion without eliciting any reaction, or destructive changes, in the invaded tissues.

The Ovarian Tumour Panel of the Royal College of Obstetricians and Gynaecologists (1983) has defined a borderline tumour as "one which shows some, or all, of the characteristics of malignancy but in which there is no stromal invasion". It will be recognised that this definition departs considerably from that employed by WHO in so far as it takes no account of the degree of epithelial abnormality: it is also in marked contrast to the position taken by those who would diagnose an adenocarcinoma even in the absence of stromal invasion. It seems, however, logical to use lack of stromal invasion as a cardinal defining feature for there is clearly a significant biological difference between invasive and non-invasive neoplasia. It is indeed tempting to equate borderline ovarian tumours with non-invasive neoplasia in other sites, such as the cervix or vulva: enthusiasm for this comparison should, however, be tempered by the fact that the stroma underlying the abnormal epithelium in a borderline tumour is, unlike that of the cervix, a component of the tumour rather than normal tissue stroma. It will be noted that all definitions of borderline tumours take into account only the histological appearances of the ovarian neoplasm: the presence or absence of extraovarian spread plays no role in the definition of borderline tumours. Even if extensive extraovarian deposits are present the ovarian neoplasm will still be placed in the borderline category if it fulfils the histological criteria for that diagnosis.

4 Serous Tumours of Borderline Malignancy

4.1 Pathology

Between 10 and 15 per cent of all serous tumours of the ovary fall into the borderline group (PUROLA 1963; HART 1977, 1981; KATZENSTEIN et al. 1978; RUSSELL 1979, 1984). To the naked eye such neoplasms closely resemble papillary serous cystadenomas but a distinction from a fully benign neoplasm is often made possible by the more luxuriant proliferation of fine papillae and by the

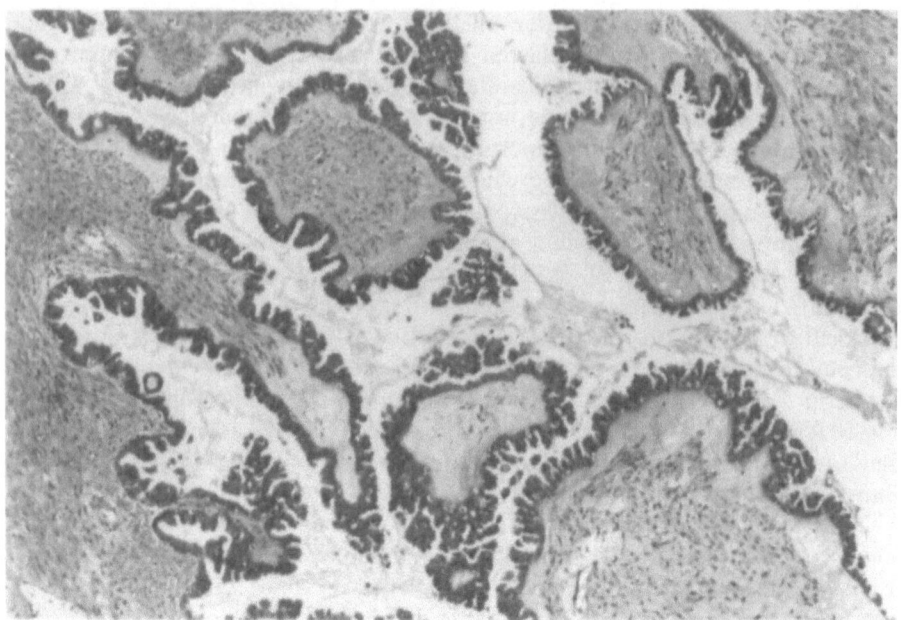

Fig. 1. A papillary serous tumour of borderline malignancy. The epithelial mantle shows atypia, multilayering and tufting but there is no stromal invasion. (H. & E. × 75)

presence of exophytic papillary excrescences on the outer surface of the cyst. Some borderline serous tumours are grossly similar to benign papillary serous surface tumours but tend ot have a more complex and dense papillary pattern.

Histologically, the borderline serous tumours are formed of rather fine, sometimes complex, branching papillae with fibrous cores. The epithelial mantle of the papillae can be clearly recognised as being of tubal type in those neoplasms with mild epithelial irregularity and atypia but with increasing degrees of abnormality, this tubal pattern is lost and the cells assume a rounded or cuboidal appearance. The epithelial component shows a variable degree of multilayering and loss of polarity and has a marked tendency to form buds or tufts (Fig. 1). These buds may break off to float freely within the cyst lumen whilst fusion or coalescence of the tips of adjacent buds often gives rise to a honeycomb appearance (Fig. 2). Nuclear crowding, atypia and hyperchromasia are of variable degree but bizarre nuclei are not seen and nucleoli are not often prominent: mitotic figures are relatively sparse and rarely of atypical form. Psammoma bodies are commonly present and are occasionally a very prominent feature.

In the vast majority of borderline serous tumours there is a sharp, clean, border between the abnormal epithelium and the underlying stroma and hence the possibility of stromal invasion can usually be readily confirmed or refuted. In some cases invaginations of epithelium to form islands within the stroma may give rise to diagnostic difficulties: such invaginations usually have smooth, rounded, rather than jagged or spiky, margins, are not associated with local stromal oedema or neovascularisation and are not accompanied by an inflamma-

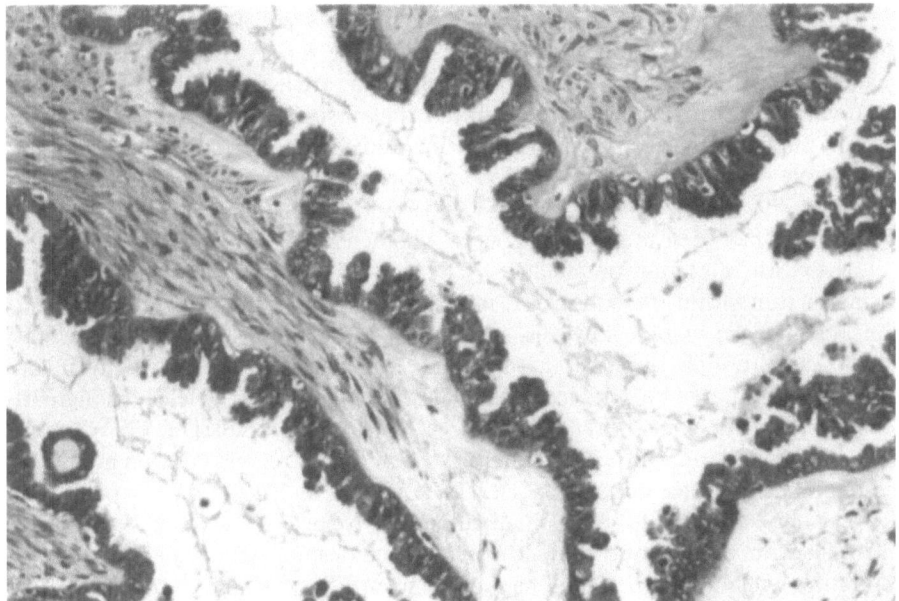

Fig. 2. Higher power view of the epithelial component of a serous tumour of borderline malignancy. (H. & E. ×190)

tory response. Keeping such criteria in mind it is usual for serial sectioning to solve the diagnostic dilemma.

Most serous borderline tumours show a remarkably constant and homogenous pattern throughout the entire neoplasm and it is relatively uncommon to find areas of clearly benign epithelium alternating, or intermingled, with epithelium showing the features of borderline malignancy. It is equally uncommon to encounter serous tumours which show a borderline pattern in some areas and a frankly malignant pattern elsewhere whilst it is exceptional for serous neoplasms to contain a melange of benign, borderline and malignant areas.

A striking feature of serous borderline tumours is their high incidence of bilaterality, this ranging in different series from 26 to 50 per cent (PUROLA 1963, JULIAN and WOODRUFF 1972; KATZENSTEIN et al. 1978; RUSSELL 1979; TASKER and LANGLEY 1985; KLIMAN et al. 1986). The variation in the reported frequency probably reflects the fact that tumour in the contralateral ovary to that containing an obvious neoplasm may not be apparent to the naked eye, being recognised only on histological examination. It is almost certain that the presence of borderline serous tumours in both ovaries represents a synchronous development of two primary neoplasms rather than metastasis from one ovary to the other: neither neoplasm exhibits any of the characteristic features of a metastatic tumour and survival rates for women with bilateral tumours are just as good as are those for patients with a unilateral neoplasm (TASKER and LANGLEY 1985; KLIMAN et. al. 1986).

A further, and often disconcerting, characteristic of borderline serous tumours is that a significant proportion, variously reported as being between 16 and 48 per cent but averaging about 35 per cent, are associated with apparent extraovarian spread at the time of initial diagnosis, this taking the form of tumour implants in the pelvic peritoneum and infracolic omentum (PUROLA 1963; AURE et al. 1971; JULIAN and WOODRUFF 1972; KATZENSTEIN et al. 1978; RUSSELL 1979; GENADRY et al. 1981; TASKER and LANGLEY 1985; KLIMAN et al. 1986). There has been much debate as to whether these peritoneal and omental lesions are true implantation metastases (SCULLY 1982) or autochthonous lesions arising in situ within the subserosal mesenchymal tissue (RUSSELL 1984). Their clinical behaviour would, however, support the latter view. Thus it is well established that although some of these lesions will progress, albeit usually in an indolent fashion, recur after a long interval or even behave as a clearly malignant adenocarcinoma (KATZENSTEIN et al. 1978; NIKRUI 1981; RUSSELL 1984) a considerable proportion will either remain stationary or regress after removal of the dominant ovarian neoplasm (TAYLOR and ALSOP 1932; GAUDRAULT et al. 1961), a fact attested to by well documented reports of women being alive and well, with no obvious evidence of tumour, despite having had peritoneal lesions for which no treatment had been given (TASKER and LANGLEY 1985; KLIMAN et al. 1986). Furthermore, it is known that extensive peritoneal lesions may be found in association with extremely small ovarian borderline tumours (McCAUGHEY et al. 1984) and with benign serous cystadenomas (RUSSELL 1984).

These clinical observations have been reinforced by histological studies, for on microscopic examination the apparent implants show a variety of patterns (McCAUGHEY et al. 1984; MICHAEL and ROTH 1986):

i. Benign lesions. These are simple tubules, sometimes cystically dilated, which may be lined by tubal-type epithelium or indifferent cuboidal cells (Fig. 3). These tubules lie below the serosa, may contain psammoma bodies and sometimes show intratubular papillary projections.

ii. Non-invasive lesions. These usually lie in mesothelial-lined cystic spaces in the subserosal mesenchymal tissue though a few form superficial surface projections (Fig. 4). These lesions are papillary and whilst some appear fully benign the appearances most commonly resemble those seen in ovarian borderline serous tumours. The cysts within which these lesions lie may sometimes be seen to be in communication with the surface. Papillary nodules, not obviously contained within a cyst, may also be seen and it is probable that these represent tumour growth which has occupied fully, and eventually obliterated, a serosal inclusion cyst. Psammoma bodies are often abundant in these non-invasive lesions which may be set in a plentiful fibrous stroma.

iii. Invasive lesions (Fig. 5). These are usually found only in the omentum and show the appearances of an infiltrating adenocarcinoma, usually, though not always, well differentiated. Invasive lesions are often associated with a desmoplastic response in the form of loose, immature fibrous tissue and may evoke a chronic inflammatory cell response.

In patients with serous borderline tumours showing apparent extraovarian spread benign lesions are present in 40 per cent, non-invasive lesions in 75

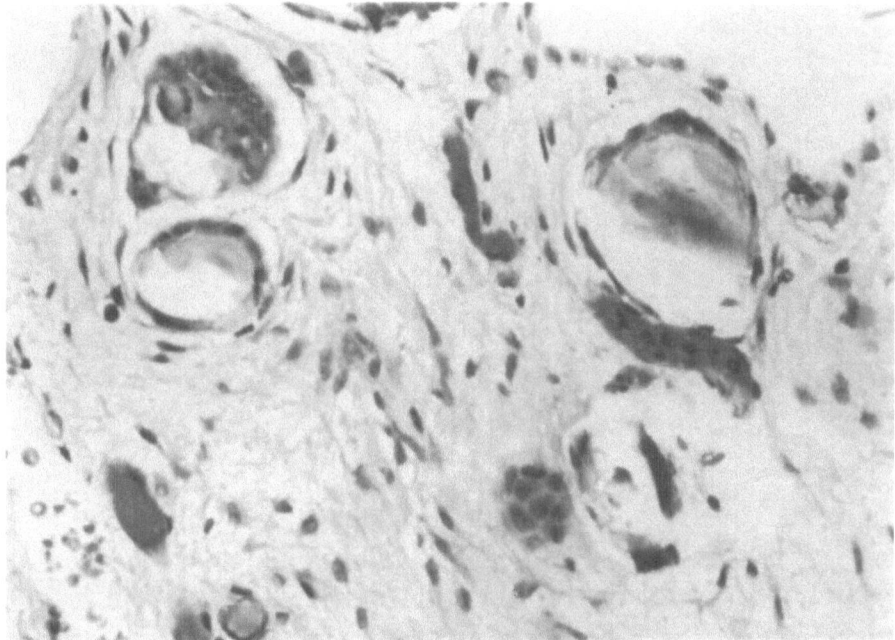

Fig. 3. Biopsy of an apparent omental implant in a patient with an ovarian serous tumour of borderline malignancy. A benign pattern is seen, only simple tubules being present. (H. & E. × 230)

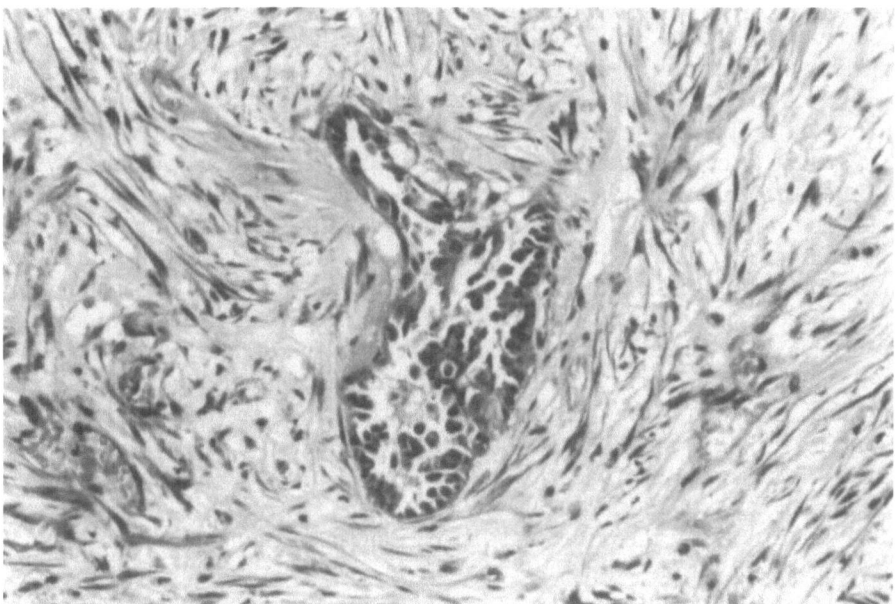

Fig. 4. Biopsy of an apparent omental implant in a patient with a serous tumour of borderline malignancy. Non-invasive lesions are present in the form of cystic spaces containing papillary epithelium showing a pattern similar to that characteristic of ovarian borderline tumours. (H. & E. × 230)

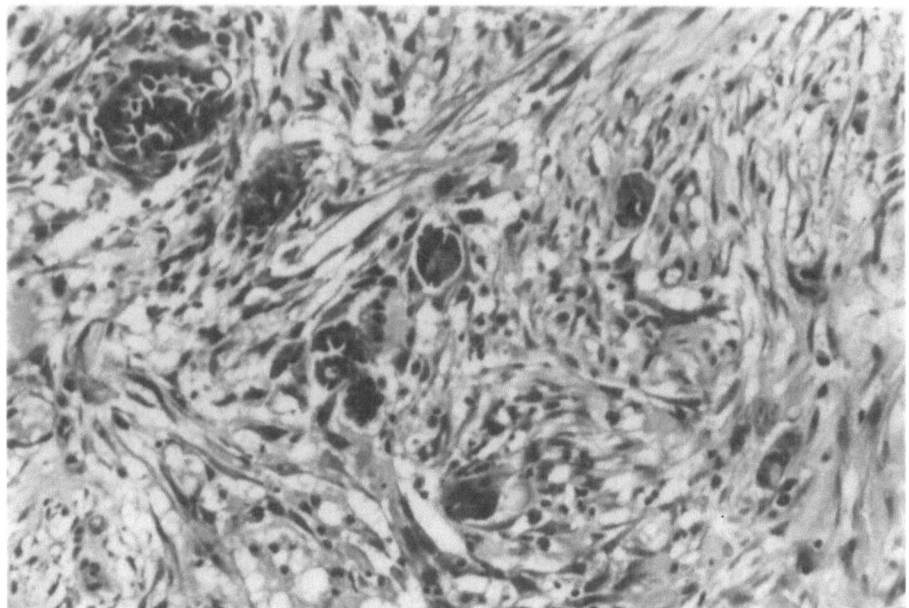

Fig. 5. Biopsy of an apparent omental implant in a patient with a serous tumour of borderline malignancy. An invasive pattern is seen with infiltrating clumps of tumour cells. (H. & E. ×230)

per cent and invasive lesions in 25 per cent. In most cases there is a simultaneous occurrence of two or three different types of lesion in the peritoneum and omentum with various permutations of the possible combinations.

These histological findings indicate strongly that the peritoneal lesions arise in situ rather than as implants from the ovarian tumour. The benign lesions correspond to the condition of endosalpingiosis (SCHULDENFREI and JANOVSKI 1962; ZINSER and WHEELER 1982) and their development bears witness to the potential for Müllerian differentiation which is a feature of the peritoneal serosa. The admixture, often an intimate one, of foci of endosalpingiosis and non-invasive lesions suggests that the peritoneal tumours arise from the benign glandular elements in the same way as ovarian serous tumours arise from cortical inclusion cysts: such lesions may progress locally to become invasive. This concept would be in accord with the clinical findings, with the fact that serous papillary carcinoma of the peritoneum can arise in the absence of an ovarian neoplasm (FOYLE et al. 1981; AUGUST et al. 1985) and with the knowledge that serous tumours of borderline type can arise in foci of endosalpingiosis within lymph nodes (FARHI and SILVERBERG 1982).

It seems unlikely therefore that the peritoneal and omental lesions found in women with serous borderline tumours are, in the vast majority of cases, true metastatic implants. This is not to deny however that serous borderline tumours can not give rise to metastases for metastatic lesions have been noted in retroperitoneal nodes (EHRMANN et al. 1980) and in extra-abdominal sites (KATZENSTEIN et al. 1978; BARNHILL et al. 1985; LAIFER et al. 1986).

4.2 Course and Prognosis

There is fairly general agreement that the overall five year survival rate for women with serous tumours of borderline malignancy is between 90 and 97 per cent, the 10 year survival rate being between 75 and 90 per cent (PUROLA 1963, AURE et al. 1971; JULIAN and WOODRUFF 1972; RUSSELL 1979; RUSSELL and MERKUR 1979; TANG et al. 1980; NIKRUI 1981; SCULLY 1982; COLGAN and NORRIS 1983; RUSSELL 1984; BARNHILL et al. 1985).

There is also a consensus that for women with Stage I disease the five year survival rate is in excess of 97 per cent with the 10 year survival rate for such patients being between 73 and 95 per cent (JULIAN and WOODRUFF 1972; AURE et al. 1971; KATZENSTEIN et al. 1978; RUSSELL 1979; SCULLY 1982; CREASMAN et al. 1982; COLGAN and NORRIS 1983; KJORSTAD and ABELER 1983; RUSSELL 1984; TAZELAAR et al. 1985; TASKER and LANGLEY 1985). Patients with Stage IIa tumours have a prognosis as good as that for women with Stage I neoplasms whilst the five year survival rate for patients with Stage IIb or III neoplasms has been reported as being between 65 and 87 per cent (KATZENSTEIN et al. 1978; JULIAN 1974; RUSSELL 1984; TASKER and LANGLEY 1985).

These survival rates should not be accepted in full without sounding a note of caution. The cited overall 10 year survival rates are based on a very small number of patients and adequate data as to the long term prognosis for women with serous borderline tumours is far from being clearly established. Furthermore, most of the quoted stage-related survival rates include a high proportion of patients treated before the introduction of adequate staging techniques. The effect of this is shown in the series of KLIMAN et al. 1986) in which before 1977, when a detailed staging technique was introduced, only 5.7 per cent of serous borderline tumours were considered to be Stage III whilst after that date 29.3 per cent of such neoplasms were allocated to Stage III. This suggests that the prognosis for Stage III borderline serous tumours may be rather better than that reported in older studies.

Two points emerge with some clarity from these reported survival rates: firstly, the overall prognosis for borderline serous tumours is considerably better than is that for well differentiated serous adenocarcinoma, thus confirming the discrete nature of these neoplasms, and, secondly, that stage, though of some clinical value, is of much less prognostic significance than is the case with frankly malignant serous neoplasms.

4.3 Treatment

The treatment of borderline serous tumours is essentially surgical. All cases should be subjected to a thorough staging laparotomy with peritoneal and omental biopsies and cytological washings of the peritoneum. The correct therapeutic approach can then be considered in (a) patients with tumour limited to one or both ovaries (Stage Ia and Ib), and (b) patients with apparent extraovarian spread.

Considering first those patients with Stage I disease. There is no debate that the optimal treatment for women, of any age, with bilateral ovarian serous borderline tumours is bilateral salpingo-oophorectomy and total abdominal hysterectomy: the same approach is also a non-contraversial treatment for women with unilateral ovarian tumours who are aged over 40 and have no wish to retain their reproductive capacity. The management of a unilateral serous borderline tumour in young women who desire to remain fertile is less well-defined though there is an increasing tendency to treat such cases by unilateral salpingo-oophorectomy (JULIAN and WOODRUFF 1972; SCULLY 1982; COLGAN and NORRIS 1983; TAZELAAR et al. 1985). This conservative approach is, of course, only valid for neoplasms which are clearly unilateral and, because it has been reported that histologically detectable tumour is present in 7 per cent of macroscopically normal contralateral gonads (WILLIAMS and DOCKERTY 1976), it is usually insisted upon that a wedge biopsy of the opposite ovary should be undertaken before conservative management of a serous borderline tumour. This view has, however, been challenged by TAZELAAR et al. (1985) who considered that wedge biopsy was of little value in carefully examined normal ovaries and documented that a negative wedge biopsy offers no guarantee of a neoplasm not subsequently developing in the examined ovary. When considering this conflict of views it has to be borne in mind that the only justification for conservative treatment is retention of fertility and that wedge biopsy of the ovary is, in itself, associated with a 14 per cent incidence of infertility. (WEINSTEIN and POLISHUK 1975). It has been recommended that after completion of her family a patient who has been treated conservatively should have a hysterectomy with removal of the remaining tube and ovary (MORROW 1981).

Surgical treatment of Stage I serous borderline tumours yields excellent results and adjuvant therapy is not indicated (SCULLY 1982; CREASMAN et al. 1982; COLGAN and NORRIS 1983; BARNHILL et al. 1985; KLIMAN et al. 1986): such therapy does not improve the prognosis and can result in subsequent acute leukaemia (O'QUINN and HANNIGAN 1985).

The management of patients with apparent peritoneal and omental implants in association with an ovarian serous borderline tumour is still far from being fully resolved. On the face of it a reasonable approach would be for a hysterectomy and bilateral salpingo-oophorectomy to be followed by individualised therapy based on the histological appearance of the peritoneal and omental lesions, those having a benign or non-invasive appearance being treated solely by surgical removal without any further therapy and invasive lesions being treated with chemotherapy.

There are unfortunately, two drawbacks to this apparently sensible course of action. The first is that progression or otherwise of abdominal disease is difficult to predict from the histological appearances of the peritoneal and omental lesions: Though, in general, invasive lesions are more likely to progress (BELL et al. 1988), this is by no means an invariable rule for such lesions may remain stationary or even regress (NIKRUI 1981; RUSSELL 1984; MICHAEL and ROTH 1986): conversely, non-invasive lesions may progress and though it has been suggested that the risk of such progression is largely restricted to those lesions showed marked cytological atypia and mitotic activity (BELL et al. 1988) this clearly implies that the atypia in the peritoneal/omental lesions should be graded, this of necessity being highly subjective.

The second drawback is that adjuvant therapy appears to be of little value in serous borderline tumours (NATION and KREPART 1986; KLIMAN et al. 1986): not only is there a very low response rate to chemotherapy but it is possible that such therapy may impair cell mediated immunity and enhance tumour growth.

It may well turn out that a more conservative approach of "watchful expectancy and masterly inactivity" should be considered for all patients with peritoneal or omental lesions and that surgical excision of tumour, rather than chemotherapy, should be the first line of attack in those women showing progressive disease (KLIMAN et al. 1986).

5 Mucinous Tumours of Borderline Malignancy

5.1 Pathology

These neoplasms, which account for 10–15 per cent of all mucinous ovarian tumours, usually present as multilocular cysts which macroscopically closely resemble a mucinous cystadenoma. Their outer surface is smooth and they usually have a multilocular appearance on section, albeit often with a finer degree of honeycombing than is the rule in benign neoplasms: focal areas of mural thickening, nodularity or endophytic papillary excrescences are often present and should raise a suspicion of the true nature of the neoplasm.

The epithelium in a borderline mucinous tumour tends to be more basophilic than is that characteristic of a mucinous cystadenoma: goblet cells are frequently present and, indeed, a majority of borderline tumours have an "enteric", rather than an endocervical Müllerian, type of epithelium. Characteristically the epithelium shows short papillary folds which often result in a serrated appearance (Fig. 6): fusion of these papillae to give a cribiform pattern is rather unusual. There are varying degrees of multilayering, loss of polarity, nuclear hyperchromatism and cellular atypia whilst mitotic figures, though seen with some frequency, are usually of normal form. Some borderline mucinous tumours have a simple pattern with a well defined epithelial-stromal junction but most have a much more complex glandular architecture with outpouchings of the epithelium and the formation of secondary cysts or glands (Fig. 7). Such features can make the assessment of possible stromal invasion more difficult than is the case with serous borderline tumours. However, this is not usually an impossible task for findings such as an irregular contour and arrangement of the glands, a focal chronic inflammatory cell infiltration and the presence of surrounding loose, immature stroma all suggest invasion rather than inclusion (RUSSELL 1979). Nevertheless, HART and NORRIS (1973) have maintained that in the absence of definite stromal invasion a mucinous tumour should be regarded as malignant, rather than borderline, if it shows a marked overgrowth of atypical epithelial cells or striking nuclear abnormalities; they also suggest that digitiform

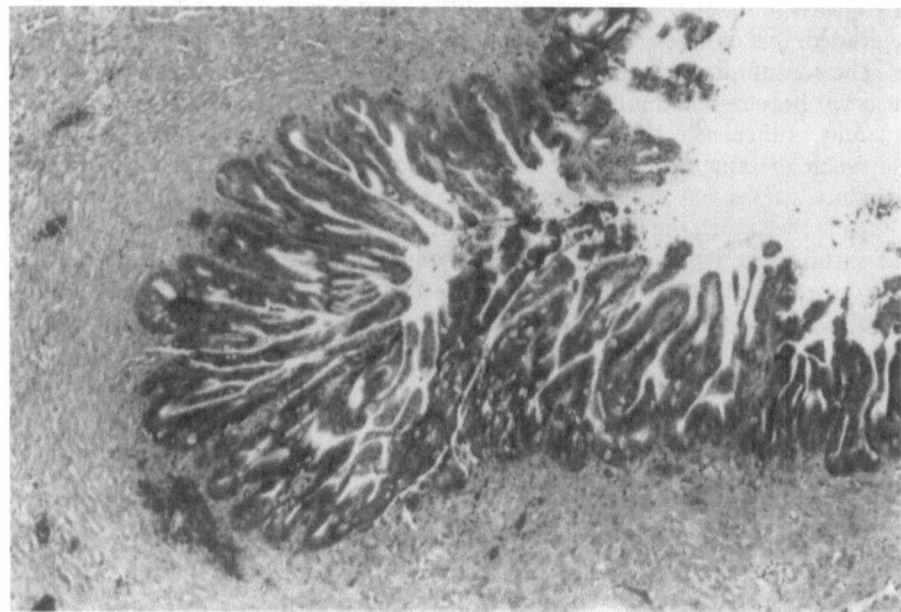

Fig. 6. A mucinous tumour of borderline malignancy. The atypical epithelium shows a serrated appearance. There is no stromal invasion. (H. & E. ×45)

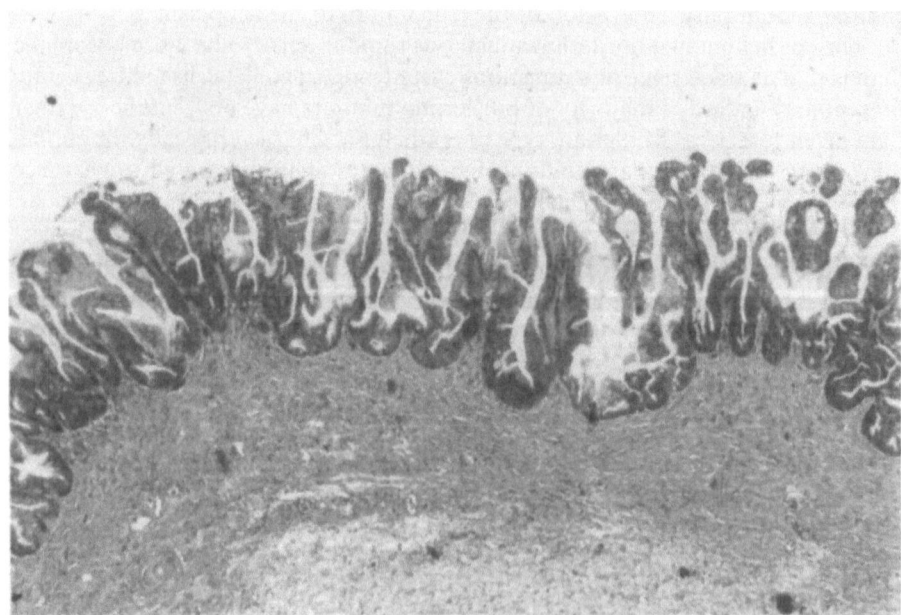

Fig. 7. A mucinous tumour of borderline malignancy. This has a complex glandular architecture which makes the assessment of possible stromal invasion difficult. (H. & E. ×75)

papillary projections of solid cellular masses which lack a stromal core should be regarded as diagnostic of adenocarcinoma and consider as malignant those tumours in which stratification of atypical epithelial cells exceeds three layers in thickness. RUSSELL (1979) has commented that "these supplementary criteria seem to add an unnecessary complication to an already difficult area which is not justified by any increased precision of prognosis": to this cogent criticism may be added the comment that a readiness to diagnose an adenocarcinoma in the absence of demonstrable stromal invasion tends to dilute the significance of invasion as a biological characteristic of malignant neoplasia and to nullify the one true defining feature of a neoplasm of borderline malignancy.

Many mucinous tumours show a stereotyped pattern of borderline malignancy throughout but a substantial proportion, probably a majority, lack the morphological uniformity of their serous counterparts and have a variety of patterns. Some show an admixture of benign and borderline areas, others borderline areas with foci of frankly invasive adenocarcinoma and yet others demonstrate, within a single neoplasm, the complete range of appearances, containing benign epithelium, areas of borderline malignancy and adenocarcinoma. This variability from area to area demands that all mucinous ovarian tumours be extensively sampled for histological examination, especially as epithelium showing the features of borderline malignancy may occur very focally in an otherwise banal tumour: similarly, foci of true adenocarcinoma within a borderline mucinous tumour can be very localised.

The incidence of bilaterality in mucinous borderline tumours is much lower than is the case with serous neoplasms, being certainly no more than 10 per cent and probably averaging about 5 per cent (HART and NORRIS 1973; RUSSELL 1979, 1984). Between 10 and 15 per cent of mucinous borderline tumours show apparent extraovarian spread at the time of initial diagnosis (AURE et al. 1971; RUSSELL 1979), this nearly always taking the form of pseudomyxoma peritonei (RUSSELL 1984), true peritoneal or omental implants being uncommon. Pseudomyxoma peritonei occurs almost invariably in association with the enteric type of ovarian borderline mucinous tumour and is characterised by the production in the abdominal cavity of large amounts of cell-poor mucus which is compartmentalised, to a various degree, by dense fibrous tissue. The condition can complicate any type of intra-abdominal mucinous neoplasm but occurs most commonly in association with mucinous borderline ovarian tumours and mucinous tumours of the appendix, two lesions which, rather confusingly, often coexist in women suffering from pseudomyxoma peritonei (SHANKS 1961). It is far from clear whether pseudomyxoma peritonei, with its continuous production of gelatinous mucus, is due to peritoneal implantation of neoplastic mucinous cells or to metaplasia, induced by mucin, of peritoneal cells into mucinous epithelium (SANDENBERGH and WOODRUFF 1977). Pseudomyxoma peritonei is often associated with pseudomyxoma ovarii (the presence of large intraovarian pools of mucus which contain clumps or strands of mucinous epithelial cells) but is not related to pre- or intraoperative rupture of a borderline mucinous tumour (HART and NORRIS 1973).

5.2 Course and Prognosis

The overall 5 and 10 year survival rates for women with borderline mucinous tumours are 87 and 85 per cent respectively (AURE et al. 1971; RUSSELL and MERKUR 1979). Patients with Stage I disease have a 98 per cent survival rate at 5 years and a 96 per cent survival rate at 10 years (HART and NORRIS 1973).

The outlook for patients with extraovarian pseudomyxoma peritonei is much more gloomy; most pursue a slow, but relentless, downhill course with a 5 year survival rate of about 45 per cent (LONG et al. 1969) and a long term survival rate which is probably no higher than 20 per cent (CARIKER and DOCKERTY 1954).

5.3 Treatment

The management of women with Stage I mucinous borderline tumours is surgical and consists, as with Stage I serous borderline tumours, of bilateral salpingo-oophorectomy and total abdominal hysterectomy for patients with bilateral neoplasms and for older women with unilateral tumours: young women with unilateral tumours can be treated by unilateral salpingo-oophorectomy and this conservative approach can, because of the low incidence of bilaterality in mucinous tumours, be embarked upon with even greater confidence than is the case when treating serous neoplasms. Adjuvant therapy has no place in the management of Stage I ovarian borderline mucinous tumours.

Patients with pseudomyxoma peritonei pose a difficult, virtually insuperable, therapeutic problem. There is no convincing evidence that either radiotherapy or chemotherapy is of any value (HART 1981) and it appears that the best approach is surgical removal of the ovarian tumour, of any definable extraovarian tumour and of as much mucus as possible, the patient's plight often necessitating repetitive surgical intervention.

6 Endometrioid Tumours of Borderline Malignancy

Endometrioid ovarian tumours which could be considered as falling into the borderline category are all of a somewhat controversial nature and this may account for the conflict of views concerning the frequency of such neoplasms, most considering them to be very rare and others regarding them as being reasonably common (RUSSELL and MERKUR 1979).

Endometrioid lesions classed as being of borderline malignancy take several forms of which one is a focal epithelial proliferation within ovarian endometriosis (Fig. 8): the proliferating glandular epithelium shows architectural and cytological atypia and the appearances resemble closely those seen in "atypical hyperplasia" of the endometrium (CZERNOBILSKY and MORRIS 1979). It is, in fact, debateable as to whether abnormalities of this type should be regarded as being hyperplastic or neoplastic in nature and all the difficulties attendant

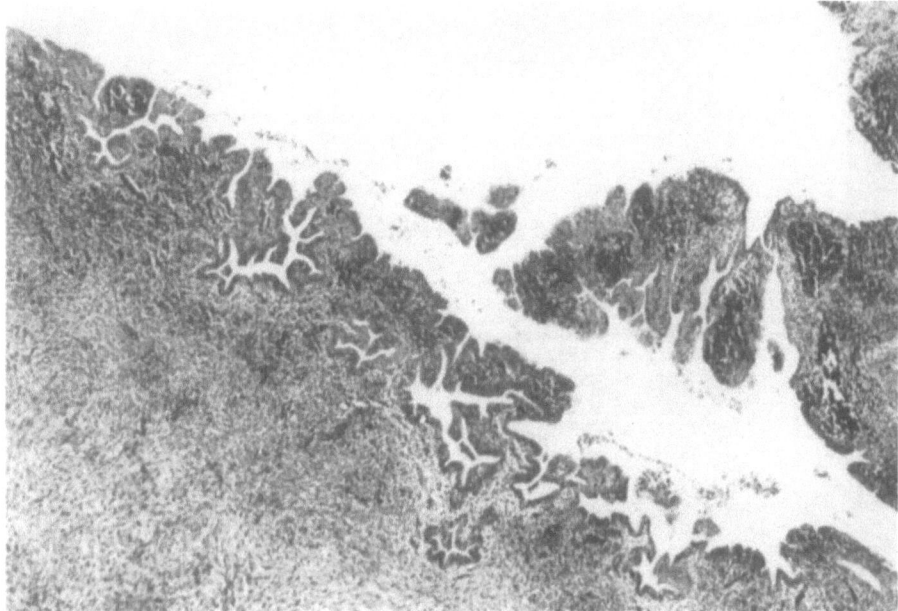

Fig. 8. An area of atypical epithelial proliferation in a fucus of ovarian endometriosis. Lesions of this type are commonly regarded, perhaps incorrectly, as a form of endometrioid tumour of borderline malignancy. (H. & E. × 45)

upon classifying such lesions in the endometrium have their exact counterpart in the ovary. It is worth noting, however, that when examining ovarian endometrioid adenocarcinomas which have clearly arisen from a focus of endometriosis it is often possible to trace a morphological continuum from the bland epithelium of the endometriotic lesion, through a pattern which resembles "atypical hyperplasia" of the endometrium, to frank adenocarcinoma. Glandular proliferation with atypia in endometriosis should be distinguished from the reactive cellular atypia which is not uncommonly seen in endometriotic epithelium but which is not associated with any epithelial proliferation.

Occasionally, ovarian cysts are encountered which have a lining epithelium of endometriotic-type cells showing all the features of malignancy but without any evidence of invasion. Whether such cysts represent true endometrioid neoplasms or endometriotic cysts showing borderline malignant change is a moot point.

The most common form of endometrioid tumour of borderline malignancy, though itself quite rare, is the endometrioid adenofibroma with epithelial atypia (KAO and NORRIS 1978; ROTH et al. 1981; BELL and SCULLY 1985). These tumours are invariably unilateral and form solid, or predominantly solid, firm grey or white masses with a smooth or bosselated outer surface. Histologically, endometrial-type glandular structures showing various degrees of atypia, such as multilayering, irregular budding and nuclear atypia, are set in an abundant fibrous stroma (Fig. 9). All such lesions are classed as "proliferative" rather

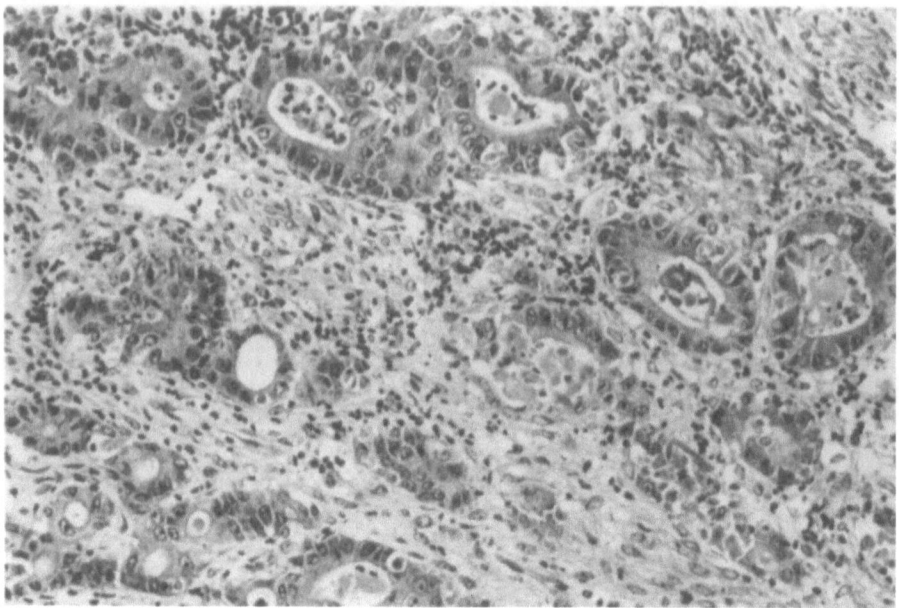

Fig. 9. An endometrioid adenofibroma in which the glandular component shows some degree of atypical proliferation. This is regarded as an endometrioid tumour of borderline malignancy. (H. & E. × 230)

than borderline by CZERNOBILSKY (1985) but BELL and SCULLY (1985) divide adenofibromas of this type into two categories: they thus recognise "atypical" endometrioid adenofibromas characterised by the presence of glands with mild to severe cytological and architectural atypia, and "borderline" lesions which contain foci of closely apposed atypical glands or epithelial islands with a cribiform pattern and low grade malignant features but without stromal invasion.

KAO and NORRIS (1978) thought that a diagnosis of adenocarcinoma arising in an endometrioid adenofibroma of borderline malignancy could only be entertained if stromal invasion was clearly present. BELL and SCULLY (1985) however, whilst accepting stromal invasion as definite evidence of adenocarcinoma, maintain that overt malignancy could be diagnosed if glands or islands of epithelial cells showing very marked atypia are present in endometrioid adenofibroma, even in the absence of obvious stromal invasion. It is a personal view that there are at present, no compelling reasons, in terms of increased prognostic precision, for subdivision of endometrioid adenofibromas with epithelial atypia: neoplasms of this type not uncommonly show a spectrum of epithelial patterns, ranging from benign to malignant, but the presence of stromal invasion, not an easy factor to assess in neoplasms of this type, should be retained as the prime prerequisite for a diagnosis of adenocarcinoma.

No instance has yet been reported of recurrence or metastasis in patients with endometrioid tumours of borderline malignancy and it appears that unilateral salpingo-oophorectomy is curative. Nevertheless too few tumours of this type have been reported for their true natural history to be fully defined.

7 Brenner Tumours of Borderline Malignancy

Tumours of this type are the subject of considerable semantic argument but nevertheless appear to be, in strictly histopathological terms, a clearly defined entity. Brenner tumours of borderline malignancy were first described as "proliferating" Brenner tumours (ROTH and STERNBERG 1971) and this term was retained in many subsequent reports (HALLIGRIMSSON and SCULLY 1972; MILES and NORRIS 1972; PRATT-THOMAS et al. 1976; CHANG et al. 1977; WOODRUFF et al. 1981). The World Health Organization classed these neoplasms, however, as Brenner tumours of borderline malignancy (SEROV et al. 1973).

Borderline Brenner tumours are usually unilateral, generally large, partly cystic neoplasms with a cut surface showing multiple locules containing clear, watery fluid. In some cases the locular lining is smooth but on others it is formed by papillary, velvety, friable tissue. Histologically, typically benign Brenner tumour is often, but not invariably, present in the more solid part of the neoplasm whilst in the papillary areas the epithelium is thrown up into multilayered folds of transitional-type epithelium which are supported by thin connective tissue stalks (Fig. 10). The appearances in these areas bear an unmistakable resemblance to a papillary transitional cell carcinoma of the bladder: cellular atypia, nuclear pleomorphism and mitotic activity are present to a variable degree but stromal invasion, which is easy to detect in these tumours, is absent.

Recently, ROTH et al. (1985) have drawn a distinction between "proliferative" Brenner tumours, which show relatively minor degrees of atypia and pleo-

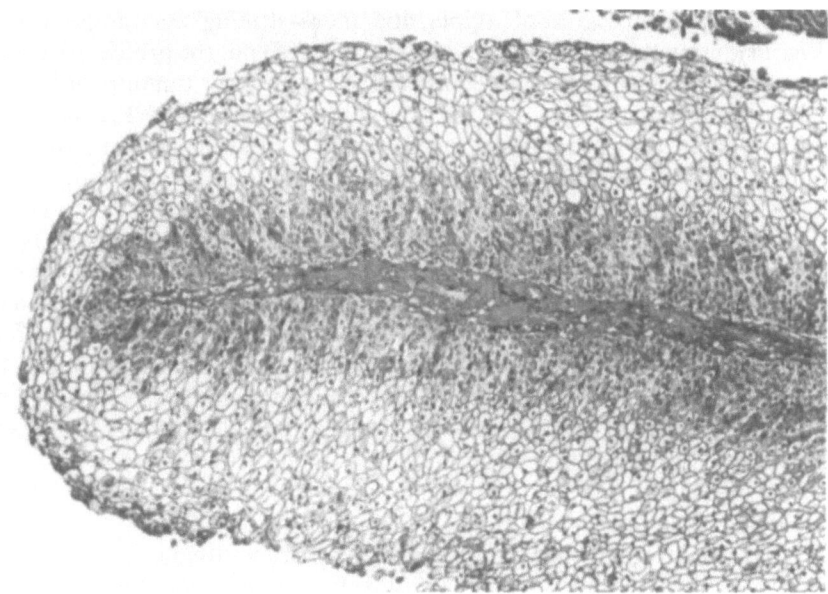

Fig. 10. The epithelial component of a Brenner tumour of borderline malignancy (proliferative Brenner tumour). In this example there is little atypia or pleomorphism. (H. & E. × 85)

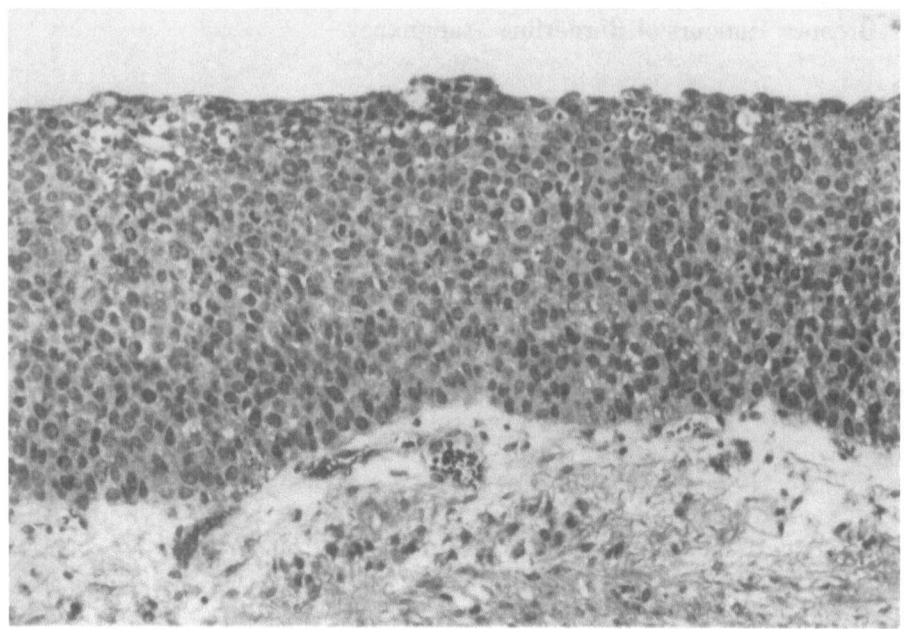

Fig. 11. A further example of the epithelial component of a Brenner tumour of borderline malignancy. This shows a failure of differentiation together with pleomorphism and atypia. (H. & E. ×175)

morphism, and "Brenner tumours of low malignant potential" which, whilst retaining the same architectural pattern, show a more marked failure of differentiation, a greater degree of atypia and more striking nuclear abnormalities (Fig. 11): using this sub-division, ROTH et al. (1985) put the proliferative Brenner tumours into a benign category and classed the Brenner tumours of low malignant potential as malignant. This subdivision of borderline Brenner tumours enforces upon the pathologist a need to make an arbitary, subjective and ill-defined division of what is, in reality, a continuous spectrum of increasing epithelial abnormality: furthermore, it has not been shown that the behaviour of, and the prognosis for, the Brenner tumours of "proliferative" type and those "of low malignant potential" differ significantly from each other. It is true that it is not uncommon for a borderline Brenner tumour to be associated with a frankly malignant Brenner tumour and that in such cases the borderline Brenner epithelium usually, but now always, shows quite marked abnormalities: this does not mean, however, that a borderline tumour showing marked atypia is, in the absence of frank carcinoma, any more likely to recur or metastasise than is one with relatively minor epithelial abnormalities. On balance, it would appear preferable to retain the single diagnostic entity of Brenner tumour of borderline malignancy.

One tumour appearing to fall into the borderline Brenner category recurred locally (McKENNA and ANSFORD 1976) whilst another metastasised to the liver (PRATT-THOMAS et al. 1976). Considerable doubt has been cast on the true nature of the latter of these two neoplasms (ROTH et al. 1985) and all other borderline

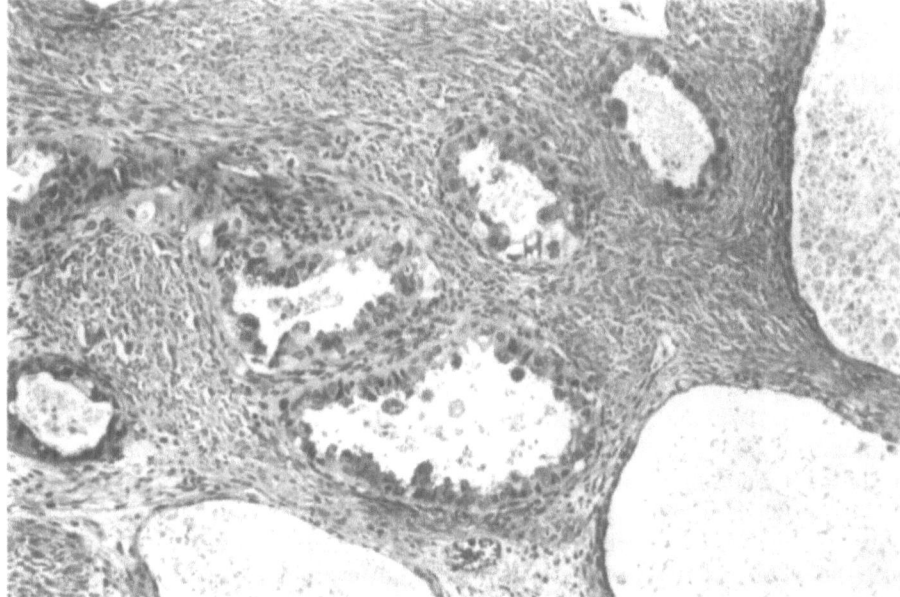

Fig. 12. A clear cell adenofibroma in which the epithelial component shows a degree of atypical proliferation. This is regarded as a clear cell tumour of borderline malignancy. (H. & E. × 100)

tumours have pursued an apparently benign course without evidence of recurrence or metastasis. Unilateral salpingo-oophorectomy would appear, therefore, to be adequate therapy for neoplasms of this type.

8 Clear Cell Tumours of Borderline Malignancy

These take the form of clear cell adenofibromas or adenocystadenofibromas in which gland-like structures lined by clear or hob-nail cells, and showing varying degrees of proliferation and aypia (Fig. 12), are set in an abundant fibrous stroma (ROTH et al. 1984). In a proportion of these neoplasms there is a transition to an invasive clear cell adenocarcinoma but in those cases in which there has been no overt invasion of the stroma there have been no instances of recurrence or metastasis.

9 Prognostic Indices in Borderline Tumours of the Ovary

Although the prognosis for patients with an ovarian tumour of borderline malignancy is generally very good, particularly for those with Stage 1 disease, the unpalatable fact remains that a few women with tumour apparently confined to the ovary will die as a direct result of their neoplasm whilst a proportion, admittedly not a very high one, of patients with extra-ovarian lesions will suffer progressive disease. A high five or 10 year survival rate may appear initially reassuring to a patient with an ovarian tumour of borderline malignancy but most women are, quite naturally, less concerned with the overall prognosis of the diagnostic group to which they belong than with their own personal chance of survival. The problem of formulating an individual prognosis, or at least of giving a clearer indication of a particular patient being one of the unfortunate minority who succumb to their disease, is a challenging one. This challenge is posed principally to the pathologist since in this group of neoplasms clinical stage is of much lesser predictive value than is the case in frankly malignant tumours, the gynaecologist thus being deprived of the most important clinical indicator of prognosis.

RUSSELL (1979) and SUMITHRAN et al. (1988) have suggested that histological grading of epithelial abnormalities in borderline tumours, in terms of the degrees of epithelial budding, multilayering, mitotic activity and cytological atypia, is of prognostic value but others have failed to confirm that histological grading offers any accurate prediction of eventual outcome (KATZENSTEIN et al. 1978; FOX 1983). In recent years there has been, however, an increasing interest in the ability of ancillary techniques, such as morphometry and flow cytometry, to identify those borderline tumours likely to be associated with a poor outlook. FRIEDLANDER et al. (1984) undertook flow cytometry of 44 borderline ovarian tumours: of these 42 showed a diploid DNA value and all these neoplasms were associated with a good prognosis. Aneuploid DNA values were found in only two cases, both of which had "invasive" peritoneal implants; one of the two patients with an aneuploid tumour went rapidly downhill and died within a few months of initial diagnosis. Clearly, these findings need to be extended but they do suggest that analysis of cellular DNA content may play a role, albeit possibly a rather limited one, in the assessment of borderline tumours.

Baak et al. (1985) made a retrospective blind morphometric study of 20 ovarian neoplasms (18 borderline tumours, one adenocarcinoma and one classified as "? borderline ? malignant"). Based on the findings in a previous study (BAAK et al. 1981) neoplasms were classed as having a "poor" prognosis if they had a high mitotic activity index together with a volume percentage of epithelium of 70 or more. Morphometric analysis of this type was able to identify, with a high degree of accuracy, the clinical outcome, for all the patients whose tumours were classed as having a "good" prognosis were alive, well and tumour-free at follow-up intervals ranging from four to 14 years whilst three tumours thought to have a "poor" prognosis (one adenocarcinoma and two borderline tumours") proved fatal within five years of initial diagnosis. Re-examination of the histology of the two borderline tumours which led to death, by pathologists aware of the outcome, failed to identify any features which would have accurately predicted the poor prognosis and thus in ovarian neoplasms of borderline malignancy the predictive power of morphometry appears to be greater than is that of unaided light microscopy. This technique, which has the further merits of consistency and objectivity, promises to be of considerable prognostic value in this group of tumours.

Although some accessory techniques do appear to have a definite role to play in the evaluation of borderline tumours, others have proved too sensitive to be of value. Thus MOUNTFORD et al. (1986) applied high resolution magnetic resonance spectroscopy to six ovarian epithelial tumours which were histologically of borderline type and found that five of the six could be designated as "malignant with a metastatic potential". The use of this technique therefore identified biological characteristics within neoplastic cells which in tumours of borderline type appear usually to be suppressed or inhibited, the technique being clearly too sensitive to be of discriminatory value in this group of neoplasms.

10 The Nature of Borderline Tumours

The true nature of ovarian tumours of borderline malignancy remains uncertain but it is apparent that, at least with the mucinous and serous neoplasms, this term is applied to two quite different patterns of neoplasia. Thus in many mucinous tumours, and in a much smaller proportion of serous tumours, there is a heterogenous pattern within the neoplasms, various combinations of benign tumour, non-invasive borderline tumour and invasive adenocarcinoma being seen within a single neoplasm. It is clear that such a tumour is one which is showing an evolving pattern, with initially benign neoplasms appearing to be undergoing a conversion to adenocarcinoma. Tumours of this type pose many questions to students of oncology for it is far from clear why overtly malignant change should occur focally in an otherwise non-invasive or benign neoplasm: even more puzzling, in view of the clonal theory of malignant neoplasia, are those tumours in which there is multifocal malignant change. Irrespective of these basic, and currently unanswerable, problems it is clear that these neoplasms showing a mixed pattern differ fundamentally from those, i.e. most serous tumours and a significant proportion of mucinous tumours, which show a homogenous pattern of non-invasive borderline malignancy throughout. A distinction has not commonly been drawn between these "static" tumours and the "evolving" neoplasms and it is possible that only the former merit placement in the "borderline" category, neoplasms with a heterogenous pattern forming a separate biological and clinical subgroup.

Despite the above caveat, many ovarian epithelial tumours of borderline malignancy show a homogenous histological pattern and are clearly not undergoing any evolutionary change. Do such neoplasms represent a discrete biological entity, are they one end of a spectrum of tumour-like atypical hyperplasia or are they simply very well differentiated, slowly growing adenocarcinomas? Dogmatic answers to these questions cannot be given but it seems unlikely that these tumours represent an extreme form of hyperplasia, in so far as a few do show spread and recurrence. On the other hand, their lack of invasiveness and their poor response to chemotherapy suggest that these neoplasms cannot be simply regarded as unusually well differentiated adenocarcinomas. Borderline tumours may indeed show a degree of cytological atypia as great, or even greater, than that found in many clearly malignant ovarian epithelial neoplasms and it does appear that the essential biological feature of borderline tumours is their lack of invasive ability, a lack that will, of course, also exclude any ability to metastasise by vascular or lymphatic pathways. This inability to invade could be due to an inherent deficiency of the tumour cells or to the host's defence reactions, the latter being presumably of an immunological nature. It is, however, very uncommon to note any significant cellular response to borderline tumours and this, together with the apparent failure of most borderline tumours to respond to chemotherapy, suggests that the specific biological features of borderline tumours are a manifestation of the inherent nature of the tumour cells and that the clinical and pathological features do not simply represent an impasse between tumour aggression and host defences. The failure to respond to chemotherapy and the slow rate of progression of borderline tumours suggest that either these neoplasms contain an unduly small population of replicating stem cells or have a normal number of stem cells that replicate at an unduly slow pace.

Some of these questions could be answered if basic oncological techniques, such as culture studies, transmission studies and clonal assays, were applied to these neoplasms and the results obtained from such studies could fundamentally alter our concepts of the biological properties of transformed cells.

References

August CZ, Murad TM, Newton M (1985) Multiple focal extraovarian serous carcinoma. Int J Gynecol Pathol 4:11–23

Aure JC, Hoeg K, Kolstad P (1971) Clinical and histologic studies of ovarian carcinoma: long term follow-up of 990 cases. Obstet Gynecol 37:1–9

Baak JPA, Blanco AA, Kurver PHJ, Langley FA, Boon ME, Lindeman J, Overdiep SH, Nieuwland A, Brekelmans E (1981) Quantitation of borderline and malignant mucinous ovarian tumours. Histopathology 5:353–360

Baak JP, Fox H, Langley FA, Buckley CH (1985) The prognostic value of morphometry in ovarian epithelial tumors of borderline malignancy. Int J Gynecol Pathol 4:186–191

Barnhill D, Heller P, Brzozowski P, Advani H, Gallup D, Park R (1985) Epithelial ovarian carcinoma of low malignant potential. Obstet Gynecol 65:53–58

Bell DA, Scully RE (1985) Atypical and borderline endometrioid adenofibromas of the ovary: a report of 27 cases. Am J Surg Pathol 9:205–214

Bell DA, Weinstock M, Scully RE (1988) Prognostic factors of ovarian serous borderline tumors with extraovarian spread. Mod Pathol 1:9A

Cariker M, Dockerty WB (1954) Mucinous cystadenoma and mucinous cystadenocarcinomas of the ovary: a clinical and pathological study of 355 cases. Cancer 7:302–310

Chang SH, Roberts JM, Homesley MD (1977) Proliferating Brenner tumor. Obstet Gynecol 49:489–493

Colgan TJ, Norris HJ (1983) Ovarian epithelial tumors of low malignant potential: a review. Int J Gynecol Pathol 1:367–382

Creasman WT, Parks R, Norris H, DiSai PJ, Morrow CP, Hreschchyshyn MM (1982) Stage I borderline ovarian tumors. Obstet Gynecol 59:93–96

Czernobilsky B (1985) Common epithelial tumors of the ovary. In: Roth LM, Czernobilsky B (eds) Tumors and Tumorlike Conditions of the Ovary. Churchill Livingstone, NewYork Edinburgh London Melbourne, p 11

Czernobilsky B, Morris WJ (1979) A histologic study of ovarian endometriosis with emphasis on hyperplastic and atypical changes. Obstet Gynecol 53:318–323

Ehrmann RL, Federschweider JM, Knapp RC (1980) Distinguishing lymph node metastases from benign glandular inclusions in low grade ovarian carcinoma. Am J Obstet Gynec 136:737–746

Farhi DC, Silverberg SG (1982) Pseudometastases in female genital cancer. Pathol Annual 17:47–76

Fox H (1983) Ovarian tumors of borderline malignancy. In: Morrow CP, Bonnar J O'Balen TJ, Gibbons WE (eds) Recent clinical development in gynecologic oncology. Raven Press, New York, p 137

Foyle A, Al-Jabi M, McCaughey WTE (1981) Papillary peritoneal tumors in women. Am J Surg Pathol 5:241–249

Friedlander ML, Russell P, Taylor DW, Tattersall MH (1984) Flow cytometric analysis of cellular DNA content as an adjunct to the diagnosis of ovarian tumors of borderline malignancy. Pathology 16:301–306

Gaudrault GL (1961) Papillary carcinoma of the ovary: report of a case with prolonged dormancy and spontaneous regression of metastases. N Eng J Med 264:398

Genadry R, Poliakoff S, Rotmensch J, Rosenstein NB, Parmley TH, Woodruff JD (1981) Primary papillary peritoneal neoplasia. Obstet Gynecol 58:730–734

Hallgrimsson J, Scully RE (1972) Borderline and malignant Brenner tumors of the ovary. Acta Pathol Microbiol Scand 80: (Suppl 233) 56–66

Hart WR (1977) Ovarian epithelial tumors of borderline malignancy (carcinoma of low malignant potential) Hum Pathol 8:541–549

Hart WR (1981) Pathology of malignant and borderline epithelial tumors of the ovary. In: Coppleson M (ed) Gynecologic oncology. Churchill Livingstone, Edinburgh London Melbourne New York, p 633

Hart WR, Norris HJ (1973) Borderline and malignant mucinous tumors of the ovary. Cancer 31:1031–1045

Julian CG (1974) Germinal epithelial neoplasia of the ovary. Clin Obstet Gynecol 17:241–257

Julian CG, Woodruff JD (1972) The biologic behaviour of low grade papillary serous carcinoma of the ovary. Obstet Gynecol 40:360–368

Kao GF, Norris HJ (1978) Cystadenofibromas of the ovary with epithelial atypia. Am J Surg Pathol 2:357–363

Katzenstein AA, Mazur MT, Morgan TE, Kao GF (1978) Proliferative serous tumors of the ovary: histologic features and prognosis. Am J Surg Pathol 2:339–355

Kjorstad KF, Abeler V (1983) Carcinoma of the ovary: borderline lesions and their therapy. In: Bender HG, Beck L (eds) Ovarian carcinoma, Gustav Fischer Verlag, Stuttgart, p 131

Kliman L, Rome RM, Fortune DW (1986) Low malignant potential tumors of the ovary: a study of 76 cases. Obstet Gynecol 68:338–344

Laifer S, Buscema J, Parmley TH, Rosenstein NB (1986) Ovarian cancer metastatic to the breast. Gynecol Oncol 24:97–102

Long RTL, Spratt JS, Dowling E (1969) Pseudomyxoma peritonei: new concepts in management with a report of the seventeen patients. Am J Surg 127:162–169

McCaughey WTE, Kirk ME, Lester W, Dardick I (1984) Peritoneal epithelial lesions associated with proliferative serous tumours of the ovary. Histopathology, p 195–208

McKenna H, Ansford A (1976) Malignant Brenner tumour. Aust NZ J Obstet Gynaecol 16:244–248

Michael H, Roth LM (1986) Invasive and noninvasive implants in ovarian serous tumors of low malignant potential. Cancer 57:1240–1247

Miles PA, Norris HJ (1972) Proliferative and malignant Brenner tumors of the ovary. Cancer 30:174–186

Mountford CE, Saunders JK, May GL, Homes KT, Williams PG, Fox RM, Tattersall MH, Barr JR, Russell P, Smith IC (1986) Classification of human tumours by high-resolution magnetic resonance spectroscopy. Lancet 1:651–653

Morrow CP (1981) Malignant and borderline tumors of the ovary: clinical features and mangement. In: Coppleson M (ed) Gynecologic oncology. Churchill Livingstone, Edinburgh London Melbourne New York, p 655

Nation JG, Krepart GW (1986) Ovarian carcinoma of low malignant potential: staging and treatment. Am J Obstet Gynecol 154:291–293

Nikrui N (1981) Survey of clinical behaviour of patients with borderline epithelial tumors of the ovary. Gynecol Oncol 12:107–119

O'Quinn AG, Hannigan EV (1985) Epithelial ovarian neoplasms of low malignant potential. Gynecol Oncol 21:177–185

Ovarian Tumour Panel of the Royal College of Obstetricians and Gynaecologists (1983) Ovarian epithelial tumours of borderline malignancy: pathological features and current status. Br J Obstet Gynaecol 90:743–750

Pratt-Thomas HR, Kreutner A, Underwood PB, Dowdeswell RH (1976) Proliferative and malignant Brenner tumors of the ovary: report of 2 cases, one with Meig's syndrome, review of the literature and ultrastructural comparisons. Gynecol Oncol 4:176–193

Purola E (1963) Serous papillary ovarian tumours: a study of 233 cases with special reference to histological type of tumour and its influence on prognosis. Acta Obstet Gynecol Scand 42, Suppl 3, 1–77

Roth LM, Sternberg WH (1971) Proliferating Brenner tumors. Cancer 27:687–693

Roth LM, Czernobilsky B, Langley FA (1981) Ovarian endometrioid adenofibromatous and cysta-denofibromatous tumors: benign, proliferating and malignant. Cancer 40:1838–1845

Roth LM, Wheeler JH, Fox H, Langley FA, Czernobilsky B (1984) Ovarian clear cell adenofibroma-tous tumors: benign, of low malignant potential, and associated with invasive clear cell carcinoma. Cancer 25:1653–1664

Roth LM, Dallenbach-Hellweg G, Czernobilsky B (1985) Ovarian Brenner tumors. I. Metaplastic, proliferating, and of low malignant potential. Cancer 56:582–591

Russell P (1979) The pathological assessment of ovarian neoplasms. II. The proliferating epithelial tumours. Pathology 11:251–282

Russell P (1984) Borderline epithelial tumours of the ovary: a conceptual dilemma. Clin Obstet Gynaecol 11:259–277

Russell P, Merkur H (1979) Proliferative "epithelial" tumours: a clinicopathological analysis of 144 cases. Aust NZ J Obstet Gynaecol 19:45–51

Sandenbergh HA, Woodruff JD (1977) Histogenesis of pseudomyxoma peritonei: review of nine cases. Obstet Gynecol 49:339–345

Schuldenfrei R, Janovski NA (1962) Dissemination endosalpingiosis associated with bilateral papil-lary serous cystadenocarcinoma of the ovary. Am J Obstet Gynecol 84:382–389

Scully RE (1982) Common epithelial tumors of borderline malignancy (carcinomas of low malignant potential). Bull Cancer (Paris) 69:228–238

Serov SF, Scully RE, Sobin LH (1973) International classification of tumours. No. 9. Histological typing of ovarian tumours. World Health Organization, Geneva

Shanks HGI (1961) Pseudomyxoma peritonei. J Obstet Gynaecol Br Emp 68:212–224

Sumithran E, Susil BJ, Looi L (1988) The prognostic significance of grading in borderline mucinous tumors of the ovary. Hum Pathol 19:15–18

Tang M, Lian L, Liu T (1980) The characteristics of ovarian serous tumors of borderline malignancy. Chinese Med J 92:459–464

Tasker M, Langley FA (1985) The outlook for women with borderline epithelial tumours of the ovary. Br J Obstet Gynaecol 92:969–973

Taylor HC, Alsop WE (1932) Spontaneous regression of peritoneal implantations from ovarian papillary cystadenoma. Am J Cancer 16:1305

Tazelaar HD, Bostwick DG, Ballon SC, Hendrickson MR, Kempson RL (1985) Conservative treat-ment of borderline ovarian tumors. Obstet Gynecol 66:417–422

Weinstein D, Polishuk WZ (1975) The role of wedge resection of the ovary as a cause for mechanical sterility. Surg Gynecol Obstet 141:417–448

Williams TJ, Dockerty MB (1976) Status of the contralateral ovary in encapsulated low grade malig-nant tumors of the ovary: Surg Gynecol Obstet 143:763–766

Woodruff JD, Dietrich D, Genadry R, Parmley TH (1981) Proliferative and malignant Brenner tumors: review of 47 cases. Am J Obstet Gynecol 141:118–125

Zinser KR, Wheeler JE (1982) Endosalpingiosis in the omentum: a study of autopsy and surgical material. Am J Surg Pathol 6:109–117

Advances in Immunohistochemistry of Ovarian Tumours

E. SAKSELA

Introduction

Immunohistochemistry has rapidly acquired an important position in present-day pathology laboratories. The expanding selection of monoclonal and polyclonal antibodies with well defined specificities has greatly increased the potentially obtainable information from routine biopsy specimens. Basically, the only limiting factors for the demonstration of the presence of any biologically significant, antigenic molecules are the specificity of the antibody on one hand and, on the other, the tolerance of the epitope(s) to the various methods required for the handling of the specimens. Appropriate characterization of the antibodies used, whether polyclonal or monoclonal is imperative. They should be thoroughly analysed for lack of cross reactions and in electrophoretic blots the antibodies should react *only* with the corresponding antigen. On the target side, overall the best results are obtained with frozen sections, fixed for instance in acetone. Alcohol or Bouin fixation followed by paraffin embedding also gives generally good results, although the long-term preservation of the material is less good. Formalin fixed and paraffin embedded material can be successfully applied in many instances although the sensitivity of detecting certain antigens including intermediate filaments can be markedly decreased. Enzyme pre-treatment of such sections can often markedly improve the results probably by degrading the cross-links that may mask the antigenic sites of many molecules. Inclusion of proper controls into each diagnostic run is of course mandatory. The technical aspects have been considered in several excellent reviews (e.g. TAYLOR 1978; LEWIS et al. 1983).

1 "Established" Markers

Some antigens can already be considered established markers since enough information is available of their behaviour in various tumor conditions and the reliability of the methods for their detection is already well established. These markers can usually also be routinely detected in formalin-fixed paraffin embedded material if some attention is paid to the selection of the antibodies used and to certain other technical details. Classical examples of such markers are carcinoembryonic antigen (CEA), alfa-fetoprotein (AFP) and human chorionic gonadotropin (HCG). Many comprehensive recent reviews already exist on the use of these established markers (e.g. KURMAN et al. 1984; KURMAN and NADJI 1985; BATTIFORA 1984) and I will treat them only briefly, concentrating on some recent interesting findings. The main cytoskeletal markers, epidermal cytokeratin, vimentin and desmin could also be included into this category but they will be discussed in more detail further below.

1.1 Alpha-Fetoprotein

One of the consistent associations is the presence of alfa fetoprotein in ovarian tumour cells as well as in the patient's serum in endodermal sinus tumours (EST). AFP is found in all types of this tumour including the polyvesicular vitelline types with characteristic Schiller-Duval bodies, in the microcystic and the alveolar glandular types as well as solid types. AFP is usually found diffusely over the tumour sections. It may also occur focally and therefore adequate sampling of the tumour is essential. Several blocks should be processed for immunohistochemistry in order to detect the AFP positive components of the tumour. AFP is the most capricious of these established markers in terms of preservation of the antigenicity of its polypeptide chains following denaturation or masking in formalin fixation. Although the quality of the antibodies in the commercially available kits has improved, it may still be necessary to make use of Bouin's fixative or, ideally, of frozen sections if careful correlations of the serum and tissue positivity are attempted or critical differential diagnostic problems exist. AFP is usually a sensitive serological marker for the existence of EST components in various types of mixed germ cell tumours or embryonal carcinomas and for the detection of these minor components, the above considerations should be kept in mind. Endodermal sinus tumours with exclusive enteric differentiation have been described (COHEN et al. 1986) as well as with hepatic differentiation (PRAT 1986) and both these types show AFP positivity.

YOUNG et al. (1984) have described a Sertoli-Leydig cell tumour in a 13-year old girl with marked serum elevation of AFP. On microscopic examination the tumour contained heterologous elements in the form of mucinous epithelium, skeletal muscle and liver cells, of which the latter component contained immuno-histochemically demonstrable alphafetoprotein. A post-operative fall of serum AFP was observed only to rise again along with the rapidly fatal recurrent course of the disease. A similar case has also been published recently by SEKIYA et al. (1985).

1.2 Human Chorionic Gonadotrophin (HCG)

Human chorionic gonadotrophin can regularly be demonstrated in hydatiform moles, chorionadenomas and chorioncarcinomas. A pure non-gestational chor-ioncarcinoma is a rare primary germ cell tumour in the ovary representing 0.6% or less of the malignant germ cell tumours encountered (VANCE and GEISINGER 1985). It does not pose usually any differential diagnostic difficulties and in this respect the regular immunohistochemically demonstrable HCG is of less importance. However, choriocarcinoma is often a component in mixed germ cell tumours, which can be verified immunohistochemically usually without difficulty in regular formalin-fixed, paraffin-embedded sections. Moreover, syn-cytiotrophoblastic giant cells (STGC) are frequently found in embryonal carci-nomas and in approximately 5% of dysgerminomas. These contain immuno-histochemically demonstrable HCG in the STGC cytoplasm. The HCG contain-ing cell component should be actively searched for in these tumours in order to alert the clinician to monitor serum HCG as a useful marker for the follow-up of the patient. The STGC morphology does not seem to be an absolute require-ment for the expression of HCG synthesis in the cells since at least two cases of reportedly pure dysgerminomas have been published which were seropositive for HCG. The hormone was found immunohistochemically in the mononuclear germinoma cell cytoplasm (ZARABI and RUPANI 1984; MULLIN and LANKERANI 1986). Occasional ovarian common epithelial tumours may also contain HCG positive cells as well as concomitant presence of the beta subunit of HCG in the serum. In one study an incidence as high as 42% of HCG positive common epithelial tumours has been reported (MOHAMBEER et al. 1983).

1.3 Carcinoembryonic Antigen

Benign, borderline and malignant mucinous ovarian tumours contain carcino-embryonic antigen (CEA). In an extensive study using a monoclonal anti-CEA antibody CHARPIN et al. (1982) found that CEA was present in 15% of ovarian mucinous cystadenomas, 80% of borderline tumours and in 100% of malignant mucinous cystadenocarcinomas. DIETEL et al. (1985) analysed the presence of immunohistochemically detectable CEA in relation to the S-phase component determined by DNA cytofluorometry and could demonstrate an increasing percentage of CEA positivity with increasing S-phase component also pointing to the correlation of CEA positivity to increasing degree of malignancy among these tumours.

The majority of benign and proliferating as well as malignant Brenner tumours are CEA positive. The staining for CEA is intense and concentrated in the cystic lumina of benign Brenner tumors but is more diffuse in the malignant and proliferating tumors. In Brenner tumours the reaction does not appear to be correlated with the degree of differentiation. All other common epithelial tumours also occasionally contain CEA. Analysis of the CEA content in the cyst fluids showed that the serous tumours were most often negative or contained only low levels of CEA when compared with mucinous tumors or endometrium (TOHYA et al. 1986). In addition, the low levels of CEA in the serous tumours were shown to include unusual CEA variants differing from the mucinous tumors containing the regular, intestinal type 200 kD molecular weight species of CEA. These findings make the immunostaining for CEA of very limited practical utility in the occasionally problematic differential diagnosis of serous ovarian tumours and mesotheliomas (SILCOCKS et al. 1986).

2 Intermediate Filaments

Intermediate filaments form an essential part of the cytoplasmic proteins in most cells. They belong to the cellular cytoskeleton, whose other components are the microfilaments (fibrils of 6 nm diameter) and microtubules (23 nm). Intermediate filaments have an average diameter of 8–12 nm and they are formed of five immunologically and biochemically different classes of subunit proteins characterizing different cell types (for recent reviews see OSBORN and WEBER 1983; WANG et al. 1985). Thus cytokeratins characterize epithelial cells, vimentin many types of mesenchymal cells, desmin is found in muscle, glial fibrillary acidic protein (GFAP) in astroglia and neurofilament triplet proteins in neural cells. In this tissue-specific expression of the intermediate filament proteins lies their usefulness in diagnostic histopathology since usually the same filament expression is also found after malignant transformation (for reviews see RAMAEKERS et al. 1983; MIETTINEN et al. 1984). Immunohistochemical analysis of the IF expression thus assists in the determination of the tissue of origin of poorly differentiated, diagnostically problematic tumours. Antibodies are by now commercially available against all classes of these subunit proteins which can be used in routinely fixed, paraffin embedded tissue sections. Still, for maximal sensitivity frozen tissues briefly fixed in acetone are preferable (NAGLE et al. 1983) and these are also suitable for rapid immunofluorescence techniques.

Characteristically, epithelia of all derivations, mesodermal, endodermal or ectodermal, express cytokeratin polypeptides as shown in Fig. 1. However, cells of the inner cell mass in an early embryo seem to be devoid of all types of intermediate filaments (JACKSON et al. 1980). As the blastocyst stage cytokeratin becomes visible at the cell borders (LEHTONEN 1985) and later the mesodermal cells as well as the parietal endodermal cells start expressing vimentin (FRANKE

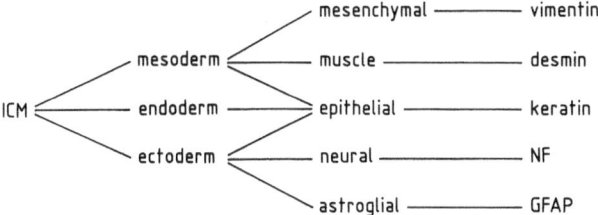

Fig. 1. Schematical presentation of the life history of intermediate filament expression in various tissues. *ICM* = Inner cell mass; *NF* = neurofilament; *GFAP* = glial fibrillary acidic protein

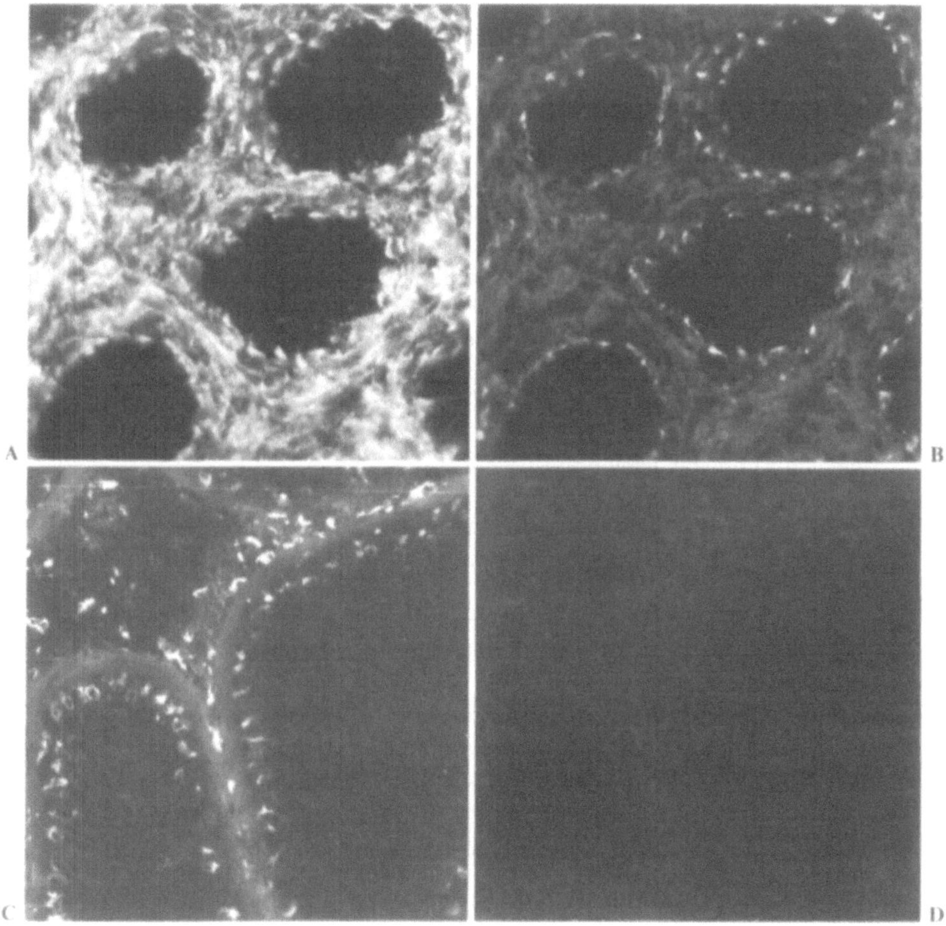

Fig. 2A–D. In fetal (**A**) and adult (**C**) testis polyclonal antibodies to vimentin show positivity in both stromal cells and in Sertoli cells of the seminiferous tubules, whereas the PKK 1 monoclonal anti-cytokeratin antibodies decorate only the Sertoli cells of the fetal testis (**B**) and the adult Sertoli cells are negative (**D**). (Courtesy of Dr. Ismo Virtanen, Department of Pathology, University of Helsinki; × 400)

et al. 1982). During embryonal development cells thus go through various stages of programmed activation and repression of the intermediate filament genes. Their expression appears thus to be linked to the so far relatively poorly understood structural and functional requirements of a particular differentiated state rather than being a cell lineage marker in a more profound meaning. The fluctuation of the intermediate filament pattern of the Sertoli cells is an illustrative example (Fig. 2). In the fetal testis the Sertoli cells express both vimentin and cytokeratin intermediate filaments. Cytokeratin filaments disappear rapidly after day 10 of the postnatal period coinciding with the hormonal maturation of the testis (PARANKO et al. 1987). The adult testicular Sertoli cells express only vimentin (VIRTANEN et al. 1986). However, in androblastomas both in testis and ovary the cytokeratin filaments again appear as shown by MIETTINEN et al. (1985). The pattern of expression of the cytokeratin intermediate filaments in these tumours thus resembles the characteristic pattern of oncodevelopmental proteins.

These considerations are of particular relevance in association with ovarian tumours. The ovary itself is derived of sex cord mesenchyme capable of both ovarian and testicular differentiation. The germ cell component is truly totipotent in its differentation capabilities. The surface epithelium is represented by the same coelomic epithelium which in the embryo gives rise to the Müllerian duct from which the oviducts, uterine body and most probably also the cervix and upper part of the vagina are derived. In this context it is thus obvious that the intermediate filament proteins in ovarian tumours cannot be used as lineage markers but rather as indicators of the various morphological differentiated states that the cellular components of the tumours can manifest.

2.1 Common Epithelial Tumours

A summary of the early findings (MIETTINEN et al. 1983) with polyclonal rabbit antibodies on the common epithelial tumours of the ovary is shown in Table 1. The findings have been confirmed with more refined monoclonal antibodies. All common epithelial tumours are cytokeratin positive and by using two-dimensional gel electrophoresis MOLL et al. (1983) have shown that of the 19 cytokeratin peptides, numbers 7, 8, 18 and 19, typical of many simple epithelia, are the main subunits expressed in these tumours. In addition, vimentin is also seen in serous tumours. It is also seen on the normal surface epithelium of the ovary. Vimentin is not usually expressed on benign serous cystadenomas but reappears in malignant serous cystadenocarcinomas (MIETTINEN et al. 1983). Double expression of cytokeratin and vimentin is also seen in mesotheliomas and thus the IF markers cannot be used in the differential diagnosis of mesotheliomas and serous carcinoma of the ovary.

Brenner tumours of the ovary express cytokeratins as shown in Table I. The cytokeratin subunit pattern in Brenner tumours resembles that seen in transitional cell papillary carcinomas of the urinary bladder (MOLL et al. 1983). These findings thus corroborate earlier suggestions on the basis of ultrastructural similarities (HAID et al. 1983) that the Brenner tumours manifest an urothelial

Table 1. Expression of intermediate filaments in ovarian common epithelial tumours[a]

	Cytokeratin	Vimentin	Desmin
Serous, benign	4/4	0/4	0/4
Serous, malignant	3/3	2/3	0/3
Mucinous, benign	3/3	0/3	0/3
Mucinous, malignant	3/3	0/3	0/3
Endometrioid carcinoma	4/4	0/4	0/4
Clear cell carcinoma	5/5	0/5	0/5
Brenner tumour	6/6	0/6	0/6

[a] MIETTINEN et al. 1983.

type of epithelial differentiation also shown by their immunohistochemical reactivity with antibodies selected for their preferred reactivity with epithelia of the urinary tract (WAHLSTRÖM and VIRTANEN 1987).

2.2 Mixed Müllerian Tumours

The malignant mixed mesodermal tumours serve as good examples of tumours in which three well established intermediate filament markers can be demonstrated in one and the same lesion (Fig. 3). The carcinomatous components stain for cytokeratins, the sarcomatous stroma with vimentin antibodies, and desmin is found in areas with smooth muscle differentiation (BONAZZI DEL POGGETTO et al. 1983). When heterologous elements occur, these express their characteristic cytoplasmic proteins (like myoglobin) in striated muscle cells. In the rare endometrial type stromal sarcomas, occasional epithelioid differentiation is seen and this can be demonstrated with immunohistochemical reactivity to cytokeratin (OKAGAKI 1986). The origin of the mixed Müllerian tumours is considered to be from clonal expansions of primitive stem cells with multidirectional differentiation capacity to various Müllerian derivatives. They thus illustrate the point made above of the role of IF proteins as differentation rather than cell lineage markers.

2.3 Sex Cord and Germinal Tumours

Normal granulosa cells of follicles of all stages have been shown to contain both vimentin and cytokeratin and they also stain for desmoplakins in accordance to ultrastructurally demonstrable desmosomes in these cells (CZERNOBILSKY et al. 1985). However, granulosa cell tumours have been repeatedly found to be cytokeratin negative and maintain vimentin reactivity (MIETTINEN et al. 1983, 1985). With desmoplakin antibodies a dotted peripheral staining is maintained (MOLL et al. 1986). These features are quite useful in the differential diagnosis of granulosa cell tumours from poorly differentiated carcinomas, which are also cytokeratin positive, and serve to separate granulosa cell tumours

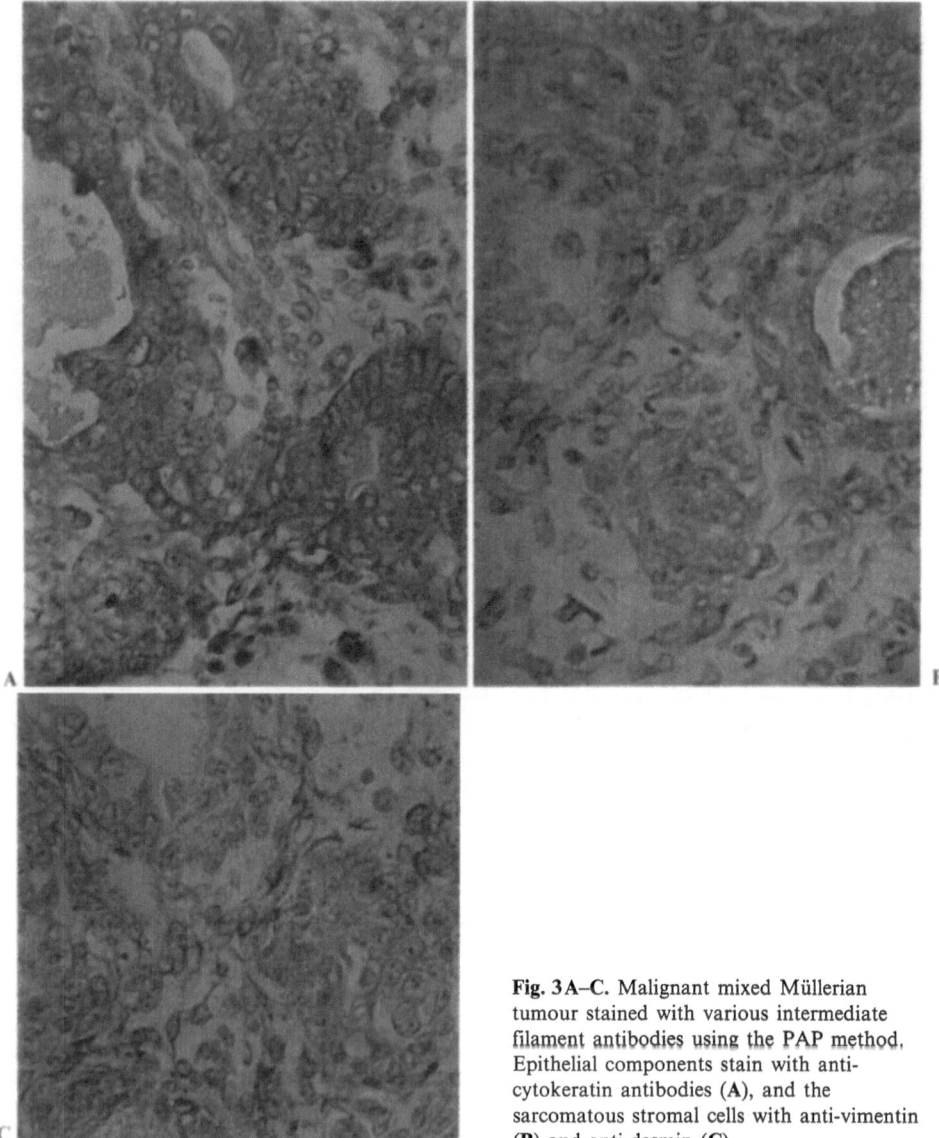

Fig. 3 A–C. Malignant mixed Müllerian tumour stained with various intermediate filament antibodies using the PAP method. Epithelial components stain with anti-cytokeratin antibodies (**A**), and the sarcomatous stromal cells with anti-vimentin (**B**) and anti-desmin (**C**)

from the desmoplakin negative pure stromal tumours. Thecomas and fibromas contain only vimentin positivity and even in the luteinized areas as well as in the non-neoplastic cortical stromal luteinized nodules no cytokeratin reactivity can be found as shown by CZERNOBILSKY et al. (1985). This study utilizing sensitive biochemical assays in addition to immunohistochemistry demonstrated a double expression of vimentin and cytokeratin also in normal corpus luteum cells and rete ovarii. There are thus at least three truly epithelial cell types in the normal ovary having the capacity to double expression of cytokeratin and vimentin which is not uncommon in cultured epithelial cells but rare in epithelial tissues. These are the ovarian surface epithelium (see above), granulosa cells and the rete ovarii epithelium (CZERNOBILSKY et al. 1985). Androblastomas have also been shown to consistently express both vimentin and cytokeratin – only one diffuse type of androblastoma without tubular structures was cytokeratin negative in an extensive study by MIETTINEN et al. 1985).

The various components of teratomas generally express their differentiation-related intermediate filament patterns. Even in poorly differentiated teratocarcinomas elements of neural differentiation have been demonstrated by the presence of glial fibrillary acidic protein (HAUGEN and TAYLOR 1984). The expansion of the immunohistochemical reagents to monoclonal antibodies against neurofilament proteins and myelin basic protein in addition to GFAP allows confident recognition of neural elements representing neurons, astrocytes and oligodendroglia, respectively, in human teratomas, which may be of clinical prognostic significance (TROJANOWSKI and HICKEY 1984). In a series of 34 germ cell tumours studied by BATTIFORA et al. (1984) even the poorly differentiated teratocarcinomas and embryonal carcinomas revealed regularly keratin positivity at least focally. However, seminomas were regularly cytokeratin negative even with the most sensitive techniques involving fresh frozen tissues or alcohol-fixed, paraffin-embedded materials tested in the study of BATTIFORA et al. (1984). This was also true for a small series of dysgerminomas as demonstrated by MIETTINEN et al. (1985). These findings thus indicate that the presence or absence of keratin by immunocytochemical methods can be helpful in distinguishing embryonal carcinomas from dysgerminomas and seminomas. It should be pointed out, however, that in a larger material of classical testicular seminomas 17 our of 41 cases showed some single cytokeratin positive tumour cells, many of which represented syncytial trophoblastic giant cells (STGC) (MIETTINEN et al. 1985). Thus more extensive series of dysgerminomas may be expected to reveal similar features.

Confirmatory evidence for the diagnosis of certain new categories of rare ovarian tumors has been obtained by the use of intermediate filament immunocytochemistry. This is exemplified by the report of KLEINMAN et al. (1984) of three apparently pure ependymomas of the ovary in young women 25 to 35 years of age. The tumours resembled common epithelial tumours of the ovary but the presence of fibrillary cytoplasmic processes and perivascular pseudorosettes alerted to the correct diagnosis confirmed by the immunohistochemical demonstration of glial fibrillary acidic protein in all cases. The use of the intermediate filament markers in the cytological diagnosis of ovarian tumours will probably form an important aspect of this clinical practice in the future. The technical feasibility of such an approach has been demonstrated by RAMAEKERS et al. (1984) by the demonstration of keratin immunohistochemically in peritoneal aspirates from patients with ovarian carcinomas.

3 Neuroendocrine Markers in Ovarian Tumours

The diffuse neuroendocrine system, or APUD system has been in the focus
of considerable research interest, particularly since the wide-spread distribution
of APUD cells has been recognized. The paracrine, tissue-level regulatory func-
tions of these neuroendocrine (NE) cells may turn out to be of major importance
once their cellular biology will be unraveled at the molecular level. The NE
cells of the APUD system have been traditionally identified by argentaffin or
argyrophil staining methods. As early as in 1938 MASSON noted the presence
of argentaffin cells in ovarian mucinous tumours but only after Fox et al. (1964)
again focused attention on the question were larger series published (KLEMI
1978; SPORRONG et al. 1981). The variety of ovarian tumour with neuroendocrine cells has been enlarged to cover a surprising diversity of tumours. These
include teratomas with endodermal components, usual carcinomas with subpo-
pulations of endocrine cells, carcinoid tumors of germ cell origin or of apparent
mesodermal derivation, atypical carcinoids and small cell (oat cell) carcinomas
(for review seen SCULLY et al. 1984).

3.1 Mucinous Tumours

Recent studies with highly sensitive immunohistochemical methods with well
characterized monoclonal reagents have confirmed the neuroendocrine nature
of at least most of the argentaffin and argyrophil cells in mucinous tumours
by demonstrating a large variety of peptide hormones and neuroregulatory
amines in these cells. In different studies reviewed by SCULLY et al. (1984) where
the simultaneous presence of argyrophilia and immunohistochemical evidence
for up to 14 different polypeptide hormones was specifically analysed in ovarian
mucinous tumours, the proportion of tumours with argyrophil cells that were
also hormone positive ranged from 20 to 100%. The variation is most likely
due to technical differences particularly in the way the tissues were prepared
for the assays. Although the peptide hormones are generally quite well preserved
in routinely formalin-fixed paraffin-embedded specimens the percentage of positive cells can be greatly increased by optimizing the fixation procedure. Also,
the techniques used for demonstration of the argyrophilia can give slightly differ-
enting results, and the role of mucin-related or glycogen-related argyrophilia
has not always been carefully controlled as pointed out by AGUIRRE et al. (1984),
who obtained a 100% correlation with argyrophilia and the presence of peptide
hormones in their careful analysis of ovarian as well as gastrointestinal tumours.
Among ovarian mucinous tumours gastrin has been identified in 3–30%, somatostatin in 2–30%, adrenocorticotrophic hormone (ACTH) in 0–34%, secretin
in 0–23%, neurotensin in 0–11%, pancreatic polypeptide in 0–7%, enkephalin
in 1% and glucagon in 0–50%. Calcitonin has not been identified in two series
where this was specifically assayed for (SPORRONG et al. 1981; AGUIRRE et al.
1984) and in the former of these studies vasoactive intestinal peptide, motilin,

beta-endorphin, insulin and substance P were not found. In contrast, serotonin was found in 15 of 16 ovarian mucinous tumours with argyrophilia by AGUIRRE et al. (1984) and in 11 of 15 similar tumours studied by INOUE et al. (1986).

3.2 Other Common Epithelial Tumours

Of the other common epithelial tumours argyrophil cells have been identified in occasional endometrioid adenocarcinomas (KLEMI and GRÖNROOS 1979) and Brenner tumours (PISCIOLI et al. 1980). FETISSOF et al. (1983) found small numbers of serotonin-immunoreactive cells among the argyrophil cell population of three benign Brenner tumours, and in a larger material of AGUIRRE et al. (1986) 11 out of 28 benign, borderline and malignant Brenner tumours contained argyrophil cells. Of these 9 reacted with antibodies to serotonin and one each to neurotensin and somatostatin. All were negative for calcitonin, gastrin, insulin, ACTH and glucagon. INOUE et al. (1986) demonstrated that 4 out of 19 endometrioid adenocarcinomas of the ovary contained argyrophil cells of the enterochromaffin type, and of these four serotonin-immunoreactive cells were found in three and somatostatin containing cells in one case.

It is well known that the ovarian Sertoli-Leydig cell tumours may contain heterologous elements in about 20% of the cases and a great majority of these are constituted of glandular or cystic structures lined by gastrointestinal type epithelium (YOUNG et al. 1982). AGUIRRE et al. (1986) studied eight such cases and the intestinal type epithelium contained in various amounts somatostatin, ACTH, gastrin, neurotensin and glucagon whereas calcitonin and insulin were not found. No clinical symptoms related to the presence of these neuroendocrine peptides were uncovered in the patients' records.

About one third of cases with primary ovarian insular carcinoid have been associated with carcinoid syndrome demonstrably relieved by removal of the tumour (ROBBOY et al. 1975). However, symptoms related to the presence of the various peptide hormones in these tumours have not been reported in the literature. No clinical carcinoid syndrome has been observed in association with pure mucinous tumours containing verified serotonin immunoreactive cells. In contrast, a clinically manifest Zollinger-Ellison syndrome relieved after removal of an ovarian mucinous cystadenocarcinoma has been reported (COCCO and CONWAY 1975), and in two subsequent cases a similar clinical course has been further associated with an immunohistochemical demonstration of gastrin in the ovarian mucinous tumor (LONG et al. 1980; JULKUNEN et al. 1983).

3.3 Other Neuroendocrine Markers

The above peptide hormones represent specific markers for neuroendocrine tumours, and require a large panel of antisera. Many authors have been looking for more general, "umbrella" markers for neuroendocrine differentiation which would cover the whole spectrum with a single or at least a limited number of immunological reagents. The neuron specific enolase (NSE) has been most notable among these broad-range markers. NSE is a useful marker applicable to routinely fixed, paraffin embedded material, which decorates most, it not all, NE cells and neoplasms. It has proven particularly useful in the differential diagnosis of poorly differentiated tumours, whose scarce content of actual neurosecretory products makes them difficult to detect with other methods. However, it has limitations since the gamma subunit of the NSE is expressed by numerous non-neural and non-NE cells. These include some subsets of lymphocytes, myoepithelial cells and even smooth muscle cells in many sites as well as certain renal tubular epithelial cells and type II pneumocytes (HAIMOTO et al. 1985; SCHMECHEL 1985; PÅHLMAN et al. 1986). NSE has been shown in ovarian carcinoids of both insular and strumal types (INOUE et al. 1985). It was not found in an ovarian mucinous carcinoid (ALENGHAT et al. 1986) nor in mucinous or endometrioid adenocarcinomas although these contained argyrophil cells with demonstrated NE activity (INOUE et al. 1985).

Another "broad-range" reagent for the immunohistochemical demonstration of neuroendocrine differentiation are antibodies against chromogranins. These are nonhormone components of the neuroendocrine granules and probably play a role in hormone storage and release (COHN et al. 1982). There is a close parallelism between the immunoreactivity against chromogranins and a positive Grimelius' staining in normal and neoplastic neuroendocrine cells (SOLCIA et al. 1986). Thus far no chromogranin immunoreactivity has been found in non-neuroendocrine argyrophil cells and related tumors, for instance most argyrophilic breast carcinomas. Chromogranin reactivity has been found in all four Brenner tumours studied containing serotonin in their argyrophil cells (AGUIRRE et al. 1986). An ovarian carcinoid tumour has also been shown to be immunoreactive with chromogranin antibodies (SOLCIA et al. 1986) but more extensive applications of this marker in ovarian tumour materials have not been published so far. Limited information is also available of the application of the natural killer cell related monoclonal antibody, HNK-1 (Leu 7), for demonstration of neuroendocrine differentiation. This antibody was described as a marker for a subset of human natural killer cells (ABO and BALCH 1981) and later found to react also with a myelin protein component of central nervous system cells (MCGARRY et al. 1983). Subsequently, it has been shown to be a marker for neuroendocrine differentiation in tumours and in NE cells (GAILLAUD et al. 1984). The NK-cell antigens detected by this antibody are relatively poorly retained in paraffin embedded, formalin fixed tissues, but it has been reported to be useful in the demonstration of neuroendocrine differentiation in tumour samples prepared this way. So, Ueda's group has shown Leu 7 reactivity in four out of 11 mucinous ovarian adenocarcinomas with argyrophil cells, in two endometrioid (out of 8) and in two out of two ovarian carcinoids (UEDA et al. 1986).

A novel marker for neuroendocrine differentiation has been recently introduced (WIEDENMANN and FRANKE 1985). This is a glycoprotein of M_r 38000 D, which has been shown to be an integral membrane glycoprotein of the presynaptic neurosecretory vesicles (WIEDENMANN et al. 1986; JAHN et al. 1985). The protein has been termed synaptophysin and it can be demonstrated in conventionally fixed, paraffin embedded tissue sections by the biotin-avidin technique in NE cells and in tumours with neuroendocrine differentiation (for review see GOULD et al. 1986). Preliminary data obtained in our laboratory indicate that it may prove useful as a marker also in ovarian tumours for the demonstration of neuroendocrine cells although in our hands more reproducible results have been obtained with frozen sections which may, after all, prove to be a requirement for the use of this marker (MIETTINEN 1987). Interestingly, it has been reported to be expressed independently of other NE markers (WIEDENMANN et al. 1986; GOULD et al. 1986) so that, for instance, a number of breast carcinomas that showed NSE immunoreactivity but failed to show other evidence of NE differentiation proved to be consistently synaptophysin-negative.

4 Monoclonal Antibodies to Tumour-Associated Antigens

The hybridoma technique for monoclonal antibodies has created a great interest in the development of tumour specific reagents with potentially unlimited supply. However, recent years have been a slight disappointment in this respect. Perhaps the most well known of these antibodies, CA 125 (BAST et al. 1983) serves as a good example of the basic problems that have been encountered. Immunization with cell suspensions and screening of the hybridomas produced with immunofluorescence or related techniques for cell surface reactivity results in most cases, as with OC 125 (KABAWAT et al. 1983a), in antibodies with carbohydrate specificities. OC 125 reacts with a high molecular weight (over 200 kD) glycoprotein structure where the epitope(s) appears to be determined by the sugars (MASUHO et al. 1984). As other cell surface glycoproteins of this type, the OC 125 antigen is shed to the cell surroundings and probably for this reason it is carried to the serum and serves as a useful serological tumour marker which may be elevated even preceding the clinical tumours (BAST et al. 1985). It was originally described as a serum marker for other than Brenner tumours and mucinous ovarian common epithelial tumours, and several studies have corroborated its clinical utility in clinical follow-up of patients. However, cross-reacting or fortuitiously similar sugar moieties are found in several other tumour types as well as in normal tissues when sensitive immunohistochemical techniques are used at the tissue diagnostic level. Up to 30% of non-ovarian cancers have been reported to be OC 125 positive (BAST et al. 1983). It stains also normal adult tissues such as epithelium of the fallopian tubes, endometrium and endocervix, mesothelial cells of the adult pleura, pericardium and peritoneum particularly in the areas of inflammation and adhesions (KABAWAT et al. 1983b). Perhaps for the later reason it has also been detected serologically in patients with various gynecological infections (HALILA et al. 1986). Consequently, OC 125 is not suitable for serodiagnosis or immunohistochemical differential diagnosis of ovarian cancer but since the serum levels in ovarian cancer patients seem to correlate with tumour regression or progression in close to 90% of patients with originally elevated values, the serum assays are useful in the monitoring of the disease.

Other published examples of the attempts to obtain ovarian cancer associated hybridoma antibodies have provided variations of the above scheme. DE KRETSER et al. (1985) described a monoclonal antibody designated OM-1 which was raised against ovarian serous cystadenocarcinoma cells. This antibody reacted strongly with primary and metastatic ovarian serous and endometrioid carcinomas but not with other types of ovarian tumour in 93 other human tumours. In normal adult tissues it decorated at least sebaceous gland cells, type II pneumocytes and placental trophoblasts so that other non-ovarian tumour reactivities may be expected when more experience is gathered. However, it is a potentially interesting antibody for the detection and possibly even for the differential diagnosis of ovarian carcinomas. OM-1 serves also as an illustrative example of the cellular biology of the glycosylated antigens detected by these methodologies. The molecule detected by the OM-1 antibody is synthetized as a 190 kD protein, cleaved to a 170 kD intracellular form which is then slowly glycosylated to a 360 kD moiety deposited on the cell surface and shed to the surrounding culture medium (DE KRETSER et al. 1986).

BHATTACHARAYA et al. (1984) have described a monoclonal antibody that appears to be at least primarily directed against determinants on ovarian adenocarcinomas. Further studies have not been reported but the same authors have described a whole panel of monoclonal antibodies against ovarian carcinoma cells or glycoprotein enriched fractions of cells. These recognize various glycoprotein surface molecules but show the limitations in terms of cross reactivity with other non-ovarian tumors or normal tissues described above (BHATTACHARAYA et al. 1985a, b). Similar findings have also been published by CORDON-CADO et al. (1985). MASUHO et al. (1984) have described an antibody designated OC 133 which shares properties with the OC 125 but detects a different glycoprotein antigen on the cells. A related monoclonal antibody designated DF3 has been suggested to enhance the sensitivity of OC 125 in the monitoring of ovarian cancer when both markers are assayed simultaneously (SEKINE et al. 1985). TSUJI et al. (1985) have suggested that the emerging patterns of reactivity in these studies might be explained by common epitopes shared by mucinous, endometrioid and mesonephroid carcinomas on one hand (Mab 43C7) and by serous and endometrioid carcinomas on the other (Mab 3C2) which are distinct for the ovarian common epithelial tumours.

At least three of a series of mouse monoclonal antibodies produced by MATTES et al. (1984) against surface antigens of ovarian cancer cells had the biochemical properties of lipids. Glycolipids will thus apparently emerge as part of the specificities detected by monoclonal hybridoma technology. This was also exemplified by the antibody (MOv 2) against cell surface glycolipids described by MIOTTI et al. (1985). No particular ovarian carcinoma type was associated with these glycolipid antigens, and the clinical or diagnostic usefulness has not been fully explored as yet. At least the MOV 2, antibody has been reported to react also with carcinomas of lung, colon, stomach and breast as well as with epithelial cells in normal lactating breast and gastrointestinal glands (TAGLIABUE et al. 1985).

So far the monoclonal technology aimed at finding specific tumour associated antigen markers has thus provided relatively little information in the immunohistological routine diagnosis of ovarian tumours. A potentially useful reagent has been described by BAILEY et al. (1986) which also serves to emphasize the capriciousness of the system based on the complexity of the glycosylation patterns of surface proteins or lipids. A monoclonal antibody was produced against a cultured human ovarian common epithelial adenocarcinoma line designated HEY. A HEY cell surface glycoprotein (40 kD) antibody (M2A) was produced which reacted with fetal but not adult testis and with seminomas and dysgerminomas but not with normal adult tissues or with other types of gonadal or extragonadal tumours. Whether this antibody will be useful in the differential diagnosis of seminomas and dysgerminoma is still unknown.

4.1 Autologous Tumour-Associated Antibodies

The idea of hunting for tumour specific autologous antibodies from immunocomplexes in ascites or cyst fluids or from ovarian cancer cell surfaces has been pursued by several groups. DOELLGAST'S group has, in a series of publications, found evidence that patients with ovarian cancer have the capacity to recognize and form antibodies against autologous tumour-associated antigens. They first studied cyst and ascites fluids from ovarian carcinoma patients which were shown to contain large amounts of various types of immunoglobulins roughly in the same molecular forms as serum immunoglobulins (KUTTEH et al. 1984). These were without detectable activity against human ovarian tumour cell lines, but apparently reacted with some cellular normal components (KUTTEH et al. 1985; LUTZ and DAWSON 1984).

However, insoluble complexes from the same sources were shown to contain membrane bound antibodies which, when eluted free, appeared to react with various autologous or allogenic ovarian tumours or tumour cell lines with immunofluorescence techniques (KUTTEH et al. 1985; KUTTEH and DOELLGAST 1986). Similar findings have been reported by QUIAN et al. (1985), and by DAUNTER et al. (1986). A similar approach starting from the immunocomplexes present in ovarian cancer ascites yielded mainly IgM containing complexes in which the antibody usually had antinuclear activity (SILBURN et al. 1984a) but when complexes with an IgG component were analysed results similar to those above were obtained (SILBURN et al. 1984b). Thus it appears that a possible way to production of diagnostically and clinically significant immunological reagents may be achieved with this strategy. So far the antigens detected have not been characterized and this is certainly a critical step before further progress can be made.

4.2 Antigens Associated with Activated Oncogens

A potentially significant approach for finding useful markers for diagnostic applications is to look for antigens encoded by activated oncogens which may play a critical role in the maintenance of the neoplastic state. Some of these oncogens have been shown to encode proteins expressed on the cell surface

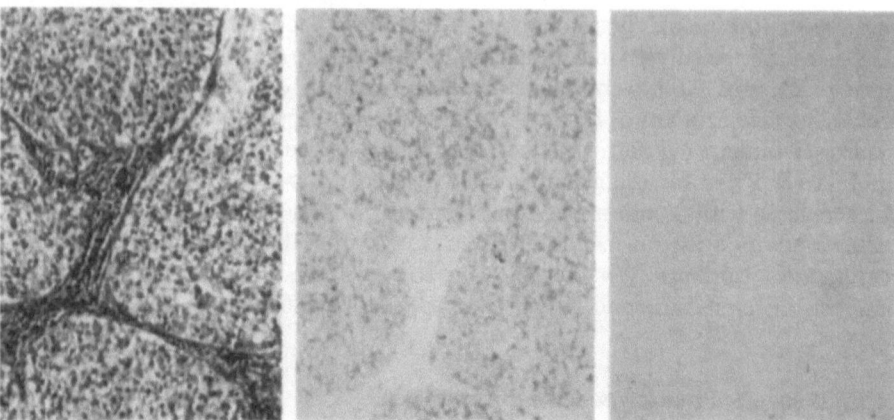

Fig. 4. Clear cell mesonephroid adenocarcinoma of the ovary stained with antibodies against a human endogenous retrovirus related undecapeptide using the PAP method (*center panel*). Routine hematoxylin-eosin stain on the left and control immunostaining with a specifically antigen-adsorbed antiserum on the right. (Courtesy of Dr. Torsten Wahlström, Department of Pathology, University of Helsinki)

and are thus possibly amenable even for therapeutic applications. The products of the erbB, fms, neu and ras oncogenes are transmembrane proteins possessing extracellular domains and one of these (neu) has recently been shown to be a target for monoclonal antibody-mediated tumor growth inhibition (Drebin et al. 1986).

Only very limited experience on the utility of oncogene related gene products in ovarian malignant tumours have been published so far. Using a rabbit antiserum to a synthetic undecapeptide deduced from a cloned human retroviral gag-gene-related DNA sequence we found a tumour-cell specific expression in all of 42 tested renal cell adenocarcinomas whereas normal kidney, 17 Wilms' tumours and a large panel of other carcinomas were negative (Wahlström et al. 1985). Subsequently we have demonstrated that ovarian clear-cell adenocarcinomas of the mesonephroid type (Fig. 4) as well as similar tumours of endometrium, cervix and the Fallopian tube were also reactive with this antibody (Wahlström et al. 1987). The expression of this apparently human endogenous retrovirus related protein is also found in developing kidneys of 18 week embryos, in placental trophoblasts and in some fetal epithelial and haematopoietic cells. The antigen thus behaves as an oncodevelopmental protein and has been useful in immunohistochemical differential diagnosis of metastatic malignancies as well as in the follow-up of patients with clear cell renal adenocarcinoma. Monoclonal antibodies produced to a synthetic peptide representing the residues 985 to 996 from the cytoplasmic domain of the epidermal growth factor (EGF) has been used in sensitive immunohistochemical analyses of human tumours involving some ovarian carcinomas (Gullick et al. 1986). High level of EGF receptor protein expression was found particularly in tumours with squamous components whereas in the adenocarcinomatous areas the staining was weak or heterogeneous. These examples serve to illustrate the potential

influence that the modern molecular biological techniques will undoubtedly
have in the development of this area of research.

Acknowledgements. I am grateful to Drs. Ismo Virtanen, Markku Miettinen and Torsten Wahlström
for their helpful comments and critical reading of the manuscript. The secretarial help of Ms. Marja-
Leena Rissanen and Ms. Outi Rauanheimo is gratefully acknowledged.

References

Abo T, Balch CM (1981) A differentiation antigen of human NK and K cells identified by a mono-
    clonal antibody (HNK-1). J Immunol 127:1024–1029
Aguirre P, Scully RE, Dayal Y, DeLellis RA (1984) Mucinous tumours of the ovary with argyrophil
    cells. An immunohistochemical analysis. Am J Surg Pathol 8:345–356
Aguirre P, Scully RE, DeLellis RA (1985) Ovarian heterologous Sertoli-Leydig cell tumors with
    gastrointestinal-type epithelium. An immunohistochemical analysis. Arch Pathol Lab Med
    110:528–533
Aguirre P, Scully RE, Wolfe HJ, DeLellis RA (1986) Argyrophil cells in Brenner tumors: Histochemi-
    cal and immunohistochemical analysis. Int J Gynecol Pathol 5:223–234
Alenghat E, Okagaki T, Talermann A (1986) Primary mucinous carcinoid tumor of the ovary.
    Cancer 58:777–783
Bailey D, Baumal R, Law J, Sheldon K, Kannampuzha P, Stratis M, Kahn H, Marks A (1986)
    Production of monoclonal antibody specific for seminomas and dysgerminomas. Proc Natl Acad
    Sci USA 83:5291–5295
Bast RC Jr, Klug TL, St. John E, Jenison E, Niloff JM, Lazarus H, Berkowitz RS, Leavitt T,
    Griffiths CT, Parker L, Zurawski VR Jr, Knapp RC (1983) A radioimmunoassay using a mono-
    clonal antibody to monitor the course of epithelial ovarian cancer. N Engl J Med 309:883–887
Bast RC Jr, Siegal FP, Runowicz C, Klug TL, Zurawski VR Jr, Schonholz D, Cohen CJ, Knapp
    RC (1985) Elevation of serum CA 125 prior to diagnosis of an epithelial ovarian carcinoma.
    Gynecol Oncol 22:115–120
Battifora H (1984) Recent progress in the immunohistochemistry of solid tumors. Seminars in Diag-
    nostic Pathology 1:251–271
Battifora H, Sheibani K, Tubbs RR, Kopinski MI, Sun TT (1984) Antikeratin antibodies in tumor
    diagnosis. Distinction between seminoma and embryonal carcinoma. Cancer 54:843–848
Bhattacharya M, Chatterjee SK, Barlow JJ (1984) Identification of a human cancer-associated antigen
    defined with monoclonal antibody. Cancer Res 44:4528–4534
Bhattacharya M, Chatterjee SK, Gangopadhyay A, Barlow JJ (1985a) Production of murine mono-
    clonal antibodies against cell-surface antigens of human ovarian carcinoma. J Surg Oncol 30:209–
    214
Bhattacharya M, Chatterjee SK, Gangopadhyay A, Barlow JJ (1985b) Production and characteriza-
    tion of monoclonal antibody to a 60-kD glycoprotein in ovarian carcinoma. Hybridoma 4:153–
    162
Bonazzi del Poggetto C, Virtanen I, Lehto VP, Wahlström T, Saksela E (1983) Expression of interme-
    diate filaments in ovarian and uterine tumors. Int J Gynecol Pathol 1:359–366
Charpin C, Bhan AK, Zurawski VR Jr, Scully RE (1982) Carcinoembryonic antigen (CEA) and
    carbohydrate determinant 19-9 (CA 19-9) localization in 121 primary and metastatic ovarian
    tumors: an immunohistochemical study with the use of monoclonal antibodies. Int J Gynecol
    Pathol 1:231–245
Cocco AE, Conway S (1975) Zollinger-Ellison syndrome associated with ovarian mucinous cystadeno-
    carcinoma. N Engl J Med 293:485–486
Cohen MB, Mulchahey KM, Molnar JJ (1986) Ovarian endodermal sinus tumor with intestinal
    differentiation. Cancer 57:1580–1583
Cohn DV, Zangerle R, Fischer-Colbrie R, Chu LLH, Elting JJ, Hamilton JW, Winkler H (1982)
    Similarity of secretory protein I from parathyroid gland to chromogranin A from adrenal medulla.
    Proc Natl Acad Sci USA 79:6056–6059

Cordon-Cardo C, Mattes MJ, Melamed MR, Lewis JL Jr, Old LJ, Lloyd KO (1985) Immunopathologic analysis of a panel of mouse monoclonal antibodies reacting with human ovarian carcinomas and other human tumors. Int J Gynecol Pathol 4:121–130

Czernobilsky B, Moll R, Levy R, Franke WW (1985) Co-expression of cytokeratin and vimentin filments in mesothelial, granulosa and rete ovarii cells of the human ovary. Eur J Cell Biol 37:175–190

Daunter B, Jaa-Kwee K, Miklosi S, Wright G (1986) Ovarian tumor antigens: preliminary histological investigation. Gynecol Oncol 23:364–370

deKretser TA, Thorne HJ, Jacobs DJ, Jose DG (1985) The sebaceous gland antigen defined by the OM-1 monoclonal antibody is expressed at high density on the surface of ovarian carcinoma. Eur J Cancer Clin Oncol 21:1019–1035

deKretser TA, Thorne HJ, Picone D, Jose DG (1986) Biochemical characterization of the monoclonal antibody-defined ovarian carcinoma-associated antigen SGA. Int J Cancer 37:705–712

Dietel M, Bodecker R, Arps H, Bahnsen J, Holzel F (1985) Borderline tumors of the ovary. New aspects on morphologic prognosis determination. Geburtshilfe-Frauenheilkd 45:213–219

Drebin JA, Link VC, Weinberg RA, Greene MI (1986) Inhibition of tumor growth by a monoclonal antibody reactive with an oncogene-encoded tumor antigen. Proc Natl Acad Sci 83:9129–9133

Fetisof F, Dubois MP, Arbeille-Brassart B, Lanson Y, Boivin F, Jobard P (1983) Endocrine cells in the prostate gland, urothelium and Brenner tumors. Immunohistological and ultrastructural studies. Virchows Arch (Cell Pathol) 42:53–64

Fox H, Kazzaz B, Langley FA (1964) Argyrophil and argentaffin cells in the female genital tract and in ovarian mucinous cysts. J Pathol 88:479–488

Franke WW, Grund C, Kuhn C, Jackson BS, Illmensee K (1982) Formation of cytoskeletal elements during mouse embryogenesis. III. Primary mesenchymal cells and the first appearance of vimentin. Differentiation 23:43–59

Gaillaud J-M, Benjelloun S, Bosq J, Braham K, Lipinski M (1984) HNK-1-defined antigen detected in uptake and decarboxylation system. Cancer Res 44:4432–4439

Gould VE, Wiedenmann B, Moll R, Lee I, Franke WW (1986) Synaptophysin: a novel marker for neurons and certain neuroendocrine cells and their neoplasms. Lab Invest 54(1):23A

Gould VE, Lee I, Wiedenmann B, Moll R, Chejec G, Franke WW (1986) Synaptophysin: a novel marker for neurons, certain neuroendocrine cells, and their neoplasms. Hum Pathol 17:979–983

Gullick WJ, Marsden JJ, Whittle N, Ward B, Bobrow L, Waterfield MD (1986) Expression of epidermal growth factor receptors on human cervical, ovarian, and vulval carcinomas. Cancer Res 46:285–292

Haid M, Victor TA, Weldon-Lipne M, Danforth DN (1983) Malignant Brenner tumor of the ovary. Electron microscopic study of a case responsive to radiation and chemotherapy. Cancer 51:498–508

Haimoto H, Takahashi Y, Koshikawa T, Nagura H, Kato K (1985) Immunohistochemical localization of gamma enolase in normal tissues, other neurons and neuroendocrine tissues. Lab Invest 52:257–263

Halila H, Stenman UH, Seppälä M (1986) Ovarian cancer antigen CA 125 levels in pelvic inflammatory disease and pregnancy. Cancer 57:1327–1329

Haugen OA, Taylor CR (1984) Immunohistochemical studies of ovarian and testicular teratomas with antiserum to glial fibrillary acidic protein. Acta Pathol Microbiol Immunol Scand (A) 92:9–14

Hood IC, Jones BA, Watts JC (1986) Mucinous carcinoid tumor of the appendix presenting as bilateral ovarian tumors. Arch Pathol Lab Med 110:336–340

Inoue M, Ueda G, Nakajima T (1985) Immunohistochemical demonstration of neuron-specific enolase in gynecologic malignant tumors. Cancer 55:1686–1690

Inoue Y, Ueda G, Yamasaki M, Inoue M, Tanaka Y, Nishino T, Saito J, Abe Y, Tanizawa O (1986) Immunohistological demonstration of peptide hormones and serotonin in ovarian mucinous and endometrial tumors with argyrophil cells. Nippon-Sanka-Fujinka-Gakkai-Zasshi 38:361–365

Jackson BW, Grund C, Schmid E, Bürki K, Franke WW, Illmensee K (1980) Formation of cytoskeletal elements during mouse embryogenesis. Intermediate filaments of the cytokeratin type and desmosomes in preimplantation embryos. Differentiation 17:161–179

Jahn R, Schiebler W, Quimeet C, Greengard P (1985) A 38000 dalton membrane protein (p 38) present in synaptic vesicles. Proc Natl Acad Sci USA 82:4137–4141

Julkunen R, Partanen S, Salaspuro M (1983) Gastrin-producing ovarian mucinous cystadenoma. J Clin Gastroenterol 5:67–70

Kabawat SE, Bast RC, Welch WR, Knapp RC, Colvin RB (1983a) Immunopathologic characterization of a monoclonal antibody that recognizes common surface antigens of human ovarian tumors of serous, endometrioid, and clear cell types. Am J Clin Pathol 79:98–104

Kabawat SE, Bast RC Jr, Bhan AK, Welch WR, Knapp RC, Colvin RB (1983b) Tissue distribution of a coelomic-epithelium-related antigen recognized by the monoclonal antibody OC125. Int J Gynecol Pathol 2:275–285

Kleinman GM, Young RH, Scully RE (1984) Ependymoma of the ovary: report of three cases. Hum Pathol 15:632–638

Klemi PJ (1978) Pathology of mucinous ovarian cystadenomas. I. Argyrophil and argentaffin cells and epithelial mucosubstances. Acta Pathol Microbiol Scand (A) 86:465–470

Klemi P, Grönroos M (1979) Endometrioid carcinoma of the ovary. A clinicopathologic, histochemical, and electron microscopic study. Obstet Gynel 53:572–579

Kurman RJ, Ganjei P, Nadji M (1984) Contributions of immunocytochemistry to the diagnosis and study of ovarian neoplasms. Int J Gynecol Pathol 3:3–26

Kurman RJ, Nadji M (1985) Immunocytochemistry of Ovarian neoplasms. In: Roth LM, Czernobilsky B (eds) Tumors and tumorlike conditions of the ovary. Churchill Livingstone, New York, p 207

Kutteh WH, Gall SA, Doellgast GJ, Allitto BA, Dawson JR (1984) Quantitation of immunoglobulins in the effusions of human ovarian epithelial neoplasms. Am J Obstet Gynecol 150:65–69

Kutteh WH, Welander CE, Homesley HD, Doellgast GJ (1985) Autologous antibodies eluted from membrane fragments isolated from the effusions of human ovarian epithelial neoplasms. I. Quantitation of antibodies. Am J Obstet Gynecol 153:124–129

Kutteh WH, Doellgast GJ (1986) Autologous antibodies eluted from membrane fragments in human ovarian epithelial neoplastic effusions. II. Tissue specificity and reactivity. J Natl Cancer Inst 76:797–804

Lehtonen E (1985) A monoclonal antibody against mouse oocyte cytoskeleton recognizing cytokeratin-type filaments. J Embryol Exp Morph 90:197–209

Lewis RE Jr, Johnson WW, Cruse JM (1983) Pitfalls and caveats in the methodology for immunoperoxidase staining in surgical pathologic diagnosis. Surv Synth Path Res 1:134–152

Long TT, Barton TK, Draffin R, Reeves WJ, McCarty KS (1980) Conservative management of the Zollinger-Ellison syndrome. Ectopic gastrin production by an ovarian cystadenoma. JAMA 243:1837–1839

Lutz PM, Dawson JR (1984) Activity of antibodies recovered from immune complexes of ovarian cancer patients. Cancer Immunol Immunother 17:180–189

Masson P (1938) Sur la présence des cellules argentaffines dans les kystes pseudomucineux de l'ovaire. Union Med Can 67:2–5

Masuho Y, Zalutsky M, Knapp RC, Bast RC Jr (1984) Interaction of monoclonal antibodies with cell surface antigens of human ovarian carcinomas. Cancer Res 44:2813–2819

Mattes MJ, Cordon-Cardo C, Lewis JL Jr, Old LJ, Lloyd KO (1984) Cell surface antigens of human ovarian and endometrial carcinoma defined by mouse monoclonal antibodies. Proc Natl Acad Sci USA 81:568–572

McGarry RC, Helfand SL, Quarles RH, Roder JC (1983) Recognition of myelin-associated glycoprotein by the monoclonal antibody HNK-1. Nature 306:376–378

Miettinen M, Lehto VP, Virtanen I (1983) Expression of intermediate filaments in normal ovaries and ovarian epithelial, sex cord-stromal, and germinal tumors. Int J Gynecol Pathol 2:64–71

Miettinen M, Lehto VP, Virtanen I (1984) Antibodies to intermediate filament proteins in the diagnosis and classification of human tumors. Ultrastruct Pathol 7:83–107

Miettinen M, Virtanen I, Talerman A (1985) Intermediate filament proteins in human testis and testicular germ-cell tumors. Am J Pathol 120:402–410

Miettinen M, Wahlström T, Virtanen I, Talerman A, Astengo-Osuna C (1985) Cellular differentiation in ovarian sex-cordstromal and germ-cell tumors studied with antibodies to intermediate-filament proteins. Am J Surg Pathol 9:640–651

Miettinen M (1987) Synaptophysin and neurofilament proteins as markers for neuroendocrine tumors. Arch Pathol Lab Med (in press)

Miotti S, Aguanno S, Canevari S, Diotti A, Orlandi R, Sonnino S, Colnaghi MI (1985) Biochemical analysis of human ovarian cancer-associated antigens defined by murine monoclonal antibodies. Cancer Res 45:826–832

Mohabeer J, Buckley CH, Fox H (1983) An immunohistochemical study of the incidence and significance of human chorionic gonadotrophin synthesis by epithelial ovarian neoplasms. Gynecol Oncol 16:78–84

Moll R, Levy R, Czernobilsky B, Hohlweg-Majert P, Dallenbach-Hellweg G, Franke WW (1983) Cytokeratins of normal epithelia and some neoplasms of the female genital tract. Lab Invest 49:599–610

Moll R, Cowin P, Kapprell HP, Franke WW (1986) Biology of Disease. Desmosomal proteins: New markers for identifcation and classification of tumors. Lab Invest 54:4–25

Mullin TJ, Lankerani MR (1986) Ovarian dysgerminoma: immunocytochemical localization of human chorionic gonadotropin in the germinoma cell cytoplasm. Obstet Gynecol 68:80S–83S

Nagle RB, Clark VA, McDaniel KM, Davis JR (1983) Immunohistochemical demonstration of keratins in human ovarian neoplasms. A comparison of methods. J Histochem Cytochem 31:1010–1014

Okagaki E Personal communication

Osborn M, Weber K (1983) Biology of disease. Tumor diagnosis by intermediate filament typing: a novel tool for surgical pathology. Lab Invest 48:372–394

Påhlman S, Esscher T, Nilsson K (1986) Expression of the gamma-subunit of enolase neuron specific enolase in human non-neuroendocrine tumors and derived cell lines. Lab Invest 54:554

Paranko J, Kallajoki M, Pelliniemi LJ, Lehto VP, Virtanen I (1986) Transient coexpression of cytokeratin and vimentin in differentiating rat Sertoli cells. Dev Biol 117:35–44

Piscioli F, Polla E, Aldovini D, Togni R, Pusiol T, Franzini M (1980) Brenner tumors: histologic types and associated lesions in the genital tract. Pathologica 72:567–572

Prat J (1986) Personal communication

Qian HN, Fenk J, Fu TY (1985) The study of antibodies and antigens dissociated from the immune complexes extracted from ovarian carcioma ascitic fluid. Gynecol Oncol 20:100–108

Ramaekers FCS, Puts JJG, Moesker O, Kant A, Huysmans A, Haag D, Jap PHK, Herman CJ, Vooijs GP (1983) Antibodies to intermediate filament proteins in the immunohistochemical identification of human tumors. An overview. Histochem J 15:691–713

Ramaekers F, Haag D, Jap P, Vooijs PG (1984) Immunochemical demonstration of keratin and vimentin in cytologic aspirates. Acta Cytol (Baltimore) 28:385–392

Robboy SJ, Norris HJ, Scully RE (1975) Insular carcinoid primary in the ovary. A clinicopathologic analysis of 48 cases. Cancer 36:404–418

Schmechel DE (1985) Gamma-subunit of the gylcolytic enzyme enolase: non-specific or neurospecific? Lab Invest 52:239–242

Scully RE, Aguirre P, DeLellis RA (1984) Argyrophilia, serotonin, and peptide hormones in the female genital tract and its tumors. A review. Int J Gynecol Pathol 3:51–70

Sekine H, Hayes DF, Ohno T, Keefe KA, Schaetzl E, Bast RC, Knapp R, Kufe DW (1985) Circulating DF3 and CA125 antigen levels in serum from patients with epithelial ovarian carcinoma. J Clin Oncol 3:1355–1363

Sekiya S, Inaba N, Iwasawa H, Kobayashi O, Takamizawa H, Matsuzaki O, Nagao K (1985) AFP-producing Sertoli-Leydig cell tumor of the ovary. Arch Gynecol 236:187–196

Senterman MK, Cassidy PN, Fenoglio CM, Ferenczy A (1984) Histology, ultrastructure, and immunohistochemistry of strumal carcinoid: a case report. Int J Gynecol Pathol 3:232–240

Silburn PA, Neil JC, Khoo SK, Daunter B, Hill R, Collins RJ, Mackay EV (1984a) Immune complexes in ovarian cancer: association between IgM class complexes and antinuclear autoantibodies in ascitic fluid. Int Arch Allergy Appl Immunol 74:63–66

Silburn PA, Khoo SK, Hill R, Daunter B, Mackay EV (1984b) Demonstration of tumor-associated immunoglobulin G isolated from immune complexes in ascitic fluid of ovarian cancer. Diagn Immunol 2:30–35

Silcocks PB, Herbert A, Wright DH (1986) Evaluation of PAS-diastase and carcinoembryonic antigen staining in the differential diagnosis of malignant mesothelioma and papillary serous carcinoma of the ovary. J Pathol 149:133–141

Snyder RR, Tavassoli FA (1986) Ovarian strumal carcinoid: Immunohistochemical, ultrastructural, and clinicopathologic observations. Int J Gynecol Pathol 5:187–201

Solcia E, Capella C, Buffa R, Tenti P, Rindi G, Cornaggia M (1986) Antigenic markers of neuroendocrine tumors: Their diagnostic and prognostic value. In: Fenoglio-Preiser C, Weinstein RS, Kaufman N (eds) New Concepts in neoplasia as applied to diagnostic pathology. Williams & Wilkins, Baltimore, p 242

Sporrong B, Alumets J, Chase L, Falkmer S, Håkanson R, Ljungberg O, Sundler F (1981) Neurohormonal peptide immunoreactive cells in mucinous cystadenomas and cystadenocarcinomas of the ovary. Virchows Arch (Pathol Anat) 392:271–280

Sporrong B, Falkmer S, Robboy SJ, Alumets J, Håkanson R, Ljungberg O, Sundler F (1982) Neurohormonal peptides in ovarian carcinoids: an immunohistochemical study of 81 primary carcinoids and of intraovarian metastases from six mid-gut carcinoids. Cancer 49:68–74

Tagliabue E, Menard S, Della-Torre G, Barbanti P, Mariani-Costantini R, Porro G, Colnaghi MI (1985) Generation of monoclonal antibodies reacting with human epithelial ovarian cancer. Cancer Res 45:379–385

Talerman A (1982) Mucinous carcinoid. In: Dallenbach-Hellweg G (ed) Ovarial Tumoren. Springer Verlag, Heidelberg, p 73

Taylor CR (1978) Immunoperoxidase techniques: practical and theoretical aspects. Arch Pathol Lab Med 102:113–121

Tohya T, Iwamasa T, Maeyama M (1986) Biochemical and immunohistochemical studies on carcinoembryonic antigen of ovarian mucinous and serous tumors. Gynecol Oncol 23:291–303

Trojanowski JQ, Hickey WF (1984) Human teratomas express differentiated neural antigens. An Immunohistochemical study with anti-neurofilament, anti-glial filament, and anti-myelin basic protein monoclonal antibodies. Am J Pathol 115:383–389

Tsuji Y, Suzuki T, Nishjura H, Takemura T, Isojima S (1985) Identification of two different surface epitopes of human ovarian epithelial carcinomas by monoclonal antibodies. Cancer Res 45:2358–2362

Ueda G, Yamasaki M, Inoue M, Tanaka Y, Inoue Y, Abe Y, Tanizawa O (1986) Immunohistochemical demonstration of HNK-1-defined antigen in gynecologic tumors with argyrophilia. Int J Gynecol Pathol 5:143–150

Vance RP, Geisinger KR (1985) Pure nongestational choriocarcioma of the ovary. Report of a case. Cancer 56:2321–2325

Wahlström T, Närvänen A, Suni J, Pakkanen R, Lehtonen T, Saksela E, Vaheri A, Copeland T, Cohen M, Oroszlan S (1985) M_r 75000 protein, a tumor marker in renal adenocarcinoma, reacting with antibodies to a synthetic peptide based on a cloned human endogenous retroviral nucleotide sequence. Int J Cancer 36:379–382

Wahlström T, Pakkanen R, Turunen O, Nieminen P, Vaheri A (1987) A multitude of malignant human neoplasms express endogenous retrovirus-related proteins which may be useful clinical tumor markers. Submitted

Wahlström T, Virtanen I (1987) Urothelial differentiation in Brenner's tumor. Submitted

Wang E, Fischman D, Liem RKH, Sun TT (eds) (1985) Intermediate filaments. The New York Academy of Sciences, New York (Annals of the New York Academy of Sciences, vol 455) pp 1–829

Wiedenmann B, Franke WW (1985) Identification of localization of synaptophysin, an integral membrane glycoprotein of M_r 38000 characteristic of presynaptic vesicles. Cell 45:1017

Wiedenmann B, Franke WW, Kuhn C et al. (1986) Synaptophysin: a marker protein for neuroendocrine cells and neoplasms. Proc Natl Acad Sci USA 83:3500

Virtanen I, Kallajoki M, Närvänen O, Paranko J, Thornell LE, Miettinen M, Lehto VP (1986) Peritubular myoid cells of human and rat testis are smooth muscle cells that contain desmin-type intermediate filaments. Anat Rec 215:10–20

Young RH, Prat J, Scully RE (1982) Ovarian Sertoli-Leydig cell tumors with heterologous elements. 1. Gastrointestinal epithelium and carcinoid: a clinicopathologic analysis of 36 cases. Cancer 60:2448–2456

Young RH, Perez-Atayde AR, Scully RE (1984) Ovarian Sertoli-Leydig cell tumor with retiform and heterologous components. Report of a case with hepatocytic differentiation and elevated serum alpha-fetoprotein. Am J Surg Pathol 8:709–718

Zarabi MC, Rupani M (1984) Human chorionic gonadotropin-secreting pure dysgerminoma. Hum Pathol 15:589–592

Subject Index

The numbers set in *italics* refer to those pages on which the respective catch-word is discussed in detail

Index of Volumes 74–77 and 79 Current Topics in Pathology